VALUES, ETHICS, LEGALITIES AND THE FAMILY THERAPIST

James C. Hansen, Editor
Luciano L'Abate, Volume Editor

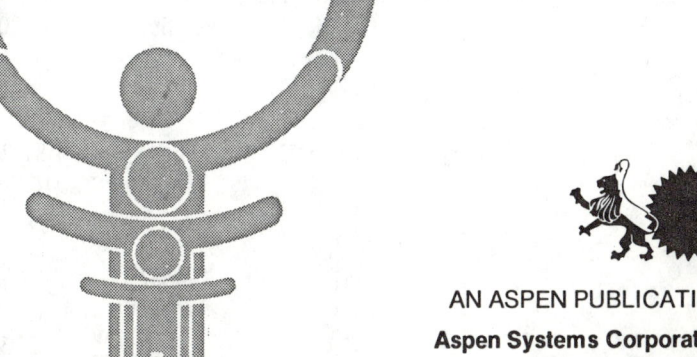

The Family Therapy Collections

AN ASPEN PUBLICATION

Aspen Systems Corporation
Rockville, Maryland
London
1982

Library of Congress Cataloging in Publication Data
Main entry under title:

Values, ethics, legalities, and the family therapist.

(The Family therapy collections)
Includes bibliographical references.
1. Family psychotherapy—Moral and ethical aspects.
2. Psychotherapy ethics. 3. Domestic relations.
I. L'Abate, Luciano, 1928- . II. Series.
RC488.5.V34   174'.2   81-20577
ISBN 0-89443-600-7   AACR2

Copyright © 1982 Aspen Systems Corporation

All rights reserved. This book, or parts thereof, may not be reproduced in any form or by any means, electronic or mechanical, including photocopy, recording, or any information storage and retrieval system now known or to be invented, without written permission from the publisher, except in the case of brief quotations embodied in critical articles or reviews. For information, address Aspen Systems Corporation, 1600 Research Boulevard, Rockville, Maryland 20850.

Library of Congress Catalog Card Number: 81-20577
ISBN: 0-89443-600-7

Printed in the United States of America

1 2 3 4 5

IN MEMORIAM

Aspen Systems Corporation

Dedicates

The Family Therapy Collections

to

Robert Curtis Whitesel
Editorial Director, Special Education

August 8, 1946 — January 27, 1982

Table of Contents

Board of Editors	vii
Contributors	ix
Preface	xi
Introduction	xv
1. Ethical, Value, and Professional Conflicts in Systems Therapy	**1**
Michael O'Shea and Edgar Jessee	
Conflicts among Therapist, Colleagues, and System Members	4
Therapist-Family-Societal Conflicts	16
Conclusion	18
2. Linear Versus Systemic Values: Implications for Family Therapy	**23**
Morris Taggart, Ph.D.	
The Epistemological Renewal	25
Linear Values and the Epistemological Challenge	29
Systemic Approaches to Values	31
The Pragmatics of Systemic Values	35
Conclusion	37
3. Counselor/Therapist Values and Therapeutic Style	**41**
Warren R. Seymour, Ph.D.	
Counselor/Therapist Values	44
Values and the Family Therapist	47
Implications for Family Therapy	57

4. **Ethical Divorce Therapy and Divorce Proceedings: A Psycholegal Perspective.**   **61**
   Florence W. Kaslow, Ph.D., and Joseph L. Steinberg, LL.B.
   One Client Unit—Two Professionals   65
   Conclusion   71

5. **Ethical Conflict in Clinical Decision Making: A Challenge for Family Therapists**   **75**
   James K. Morrison, Ph.D., Bruce Layton, Ph.D., and Joan Newman, Ph.D.
   Ethical Issues within the General Clinical Field   77
   Ethical Issues and Family Therapy   80
   A Survey of Ethical Conflicts among Clinicians   81

6. **Ignorance of the Law Is No Excuse**   **87**
   Barton E. Bernstein, M.L.A., J.D.
   The Elderly and Terminally Ill   90
   Serving the Survivor   92
   Cohabitation   93
   The Child as a Witness   94
   The Premarital Agreement   96
   Divorce/Family Counseling   97

7. **Issues in Family Law: Implications for Therapists**   **103**
   R. Barry Ruback, J.D., Ph.D.
   The Legal Process   106
   History and Present Context of Family Law   107
   Law of Marriage   107
   Dissolution of Marriage   108
   Establishing the Parent-Child Relationship   110
   Parents' Rights and Duties to Children   111
   Child Custody in Divorce   112
   Juvenile Justice   116
   Role of the Family Therapist in Legal Proceedings   117
   Implications for the Family Therapist   118

8. **The Regulation of Marital and Family Therapy**   **125**
   Michael Sporakowski, Ph.D.
   Regulation of Marital and Family Therapy   128
   Significance to the Practitioner   129
   A Broader Perspective   132
   Conclusion   133

Board of Editors

Editor
JAMES C. HANSEN
State University of New York at Buffalo
Buffalo, New York

JAMES F. ALEXANDER
University of Utah
Salt Lake City, Utah

CAROLYN L. ATTNEAVE
University of Washington
Seattle, Washington

JOHN ELDERKIN BELL
Stanford University
Palo Alto, California

HOLLIS A. EDWARDS
Toronto East General Hospital
Toronto Family Therapy Institute
Toronto, Ontario, Canada

NATHAN B. EPSTEIN
Brown University
Butler Hospital
Providence, Rhode Island

ALAN S. GURMAN
University of Wisconsin Medical School
Madison, Wisconsin

JOHN HOWELLS
Institute of Family Psychiatry
Ipswich, England

FLORENCE W. KASLOW
Kaslow Associates, P.A.
West Palm Beach, Florida

DAVID P. KNISKERN
University of Cincinnati
College of Medicine
Central Psychiatric Clinic
Cincinnati, Ohio

LUCIANO L'ABATE
Georgia State University
Atlanta, Georgia

KITTY LAPERRIERE
Ackerman Institute for Family Therapy
Columbia University School of Medicine
New York, New York

ARTHUR MANDELBAUM
The Menninger Foundation
Topeka, Kansas

AUGUSTUS Y. NAPIER
The Family Workshop
Atlanta, Georgia

Board of Editors
(continued)

DAVID H. OLSON
University of Minnesota
St. Paul, Minnesota

VIRGINIA M. SATIR
ANTERRA, Inc.
Menlo Park, California

RODNEY J. SHAPIRO
Veterans Administration Medical
Center
San Francisco, California

JUDITH S. WALLERSTEIN
Center for the Family in
Transition
Corte Madera, California

CARL A. WHITAKER
University of Wisconsin-Madison
Madison, Wisconsin

ROBERT HENLEY WOODY
University of Nebraska at Omaha
Omaha, Nebraska

Contributors

Volume Editor
LUCIANO L'ABATE
Georgia State University
Atlanta, Georgia

BARTON E. BERNSTEIN
Southwestern Medical School
Dallas, Texas

MICHAEL O'SHEA
Texas Medical Center
Houston, Texas

EDGAR JESSEE
Institute for Juvenile Research
Chicago, Illinois

R. BARRY RUBACK
Georgia State University
Atlanta, Georgia

FLORENCE W. KASLOW
Kaslow Associates, P.A.
West Palm Beach, Florida

WARREN R. SEYMOUR
University of Missouri-Columbia
Columbia, Missouri

BRUCE LAYTON
U.S. General Accounting Office
Washington, D.C.

MICHAEL J. SPORAKOWSKI
Virginia Polytechnic Institute and
State University
Blacksburg, Virginia

JAMES K. MORRISON
Albany Medical College
Albany, New York

JOSEPH L. STEINBERG
University of Connecticut
Hartford, Connecticut

JOAN NEWMAN
State University of New York at
Albany
Albany, New York

MORRIS TAGGART
Houston-Galveston Family
Institute
Houston, Texas

Preface

Family therapy has developed and expanded considerably from the early 1950s when a few pioneering therapists worked with families and several individuals investigated family interactions. These experiences have grown into general theories of family interrelations, and a field of family therapy has evolved. Various theoretical approaches have developed, process and outcome studies have been conducted, and a burgeoning literature has emerged. With this rapid growth there is a growing professional concern and responsibility to assist in the education of family therapists by providing them with integrated information.

Although theory, research, and publications in family therapy are abundant, no single source exists which provides the practical applications that can be employed by the professional. *The Family Therapy Collections* will serve as the source of information for both the student and practicing professional by gathering, synthesizing, and applying the research and literature of the field. The *Collections* will not publish esoteric research or rehash conceptual articles; it will provide a synthesis of significant topics in the field that meet the needs of the practitioner. The *Collections* will provide a forum that not only translates theory and research into practice but also presents perspectives on the status, issues, and trends in a manner that stimulates advances and innovations in the field of family therapy.

The purpose of the *Collections* is to provide professionals with a continuity publication that reviews topics of current and specific research and translates theoretical concepts into practical application. Each volume will consist of a collection of articles that provide in-depth coverage of a single significant aspect of family therapy. The series of volumes will serve as a collection of topics in family therapy. The term *Collections* has been carefully chosen and is plural to reflect the collective nature of each volume as well as the collective nature of the series, viewed as a whole body of professional practice literature.

All articles will be authored by practicing professionals in family therapy. The literature will be analyzed with an emphasis on the implications for practice. The emphasis on meaningful application by practitioners does not mean that it will be a how-to-do-it publication; rather, we will strive to present concepts and findings in a manner that thoughtful professionals can then apply. Original research will be published if it is clearly focused on a family therapy issue, meets standards of experimental design and data analysis, and presents findings with clear implications for practice that are fully discussed.

Each volume in the series will have a volume editor. The field of family therapy is too broad for a single individual to possess the knowledge and network of professional acquaintances necessary to edit each topic issue competently. Volume editors will be responsible for assisting in topic development and inviting people with expertise in specific areas to submit articles. Through this procedure the *Collections* can present an integrated coverage of the topic by leading professionals in that area.

The editorial board selected to evaluate manuscripts submitted to the publication and invited by the editorial staff includes family therapy professionals representing a wide variety of disciplines. Some are noted for their theoretical developments, others for their research contributions, but all are recognized as having distinguished careers in the field. With an editorial board so constituted, we hope to provide fair review of all manuscripts and accurate, cross-disciplinary content.

THE INAUGURAL VOLUME

This first volume of *The Family Therapy Collections* addresses an area that is of great professional concern. Irrespective of one's theoretical approach or specific intervention techniques, addressing the values, ethics, and legalities affecting the family therapist is paramount.

Luciano L'Abate is the editor for this volume. He is Professor of Psychology at Georgia State University where he specializes in training family therapists. The combination of his training responsibilities and his own work as a family therapist provides him an excellent perspective to focus on the issues of values, ethics, and legalities as they affect the family therapist.

Values are the personal criteria that include ideals, goals, norms, and standards of behavior that are reflected in the activities and decisions that each person makes. A therapist's beliefs can certainly influence his or her behavior in family therapy. Therapists need to be aware not only of their own values but also those of the family and the possibility of conflicts between the two. In the area of family therapy, it has become apparent that not only are personal values involved but the professional values inherent in systems theory may cause various professional conflicts, as well. Clearly this area requires considerable thought to ensure professional integrity.

Ethics are suggested standards of behavior based on a consensus of professional values. Family therapists have attempted to translate as many as possible into structured expectations of behavior. Ethical standards are guidelines; however, it seems that therapists continually face situations that cause conflict and require decision making on their part. The more ethical topics are considered, the better one is prepared when problem situations arise.

In some cases there is a close relationship between ethics and legalities. The potential for legal action is increasing, and it is important for family therapists to be aware of their legal status. Therapists certainly can improve their services by becoming more aware of the laws that affect family problems.

The topic seems particularly appropriate for the first collection. It is clear that professional practice is based on therapists' knowledge and the integration of these concepts into their behavior.

James C. Hansen
Editor

Introduction

The issues of values, ethics, and legalities are timely topics in family therapy. No longer can marriage and family therapists claim neutrality or irrelevance. It is important for therapists to be aware of their personal and professional values and ethics as well as their potential impact during therapy. Likewise, therapists need to be knowledgeable of the basic principles of family law to most effectively assist their clientele. Try to define and distinguish among ethical, professional, moral, and legal. Once this discrimination is made, relate these distinctions to your personal and professional life. How can neutrality be maintained? Even more to the point, how can ignorance or disinterest be maintained? One cannot practice therapy without being touched by moral, legal, professional, and ethical issues. It is humanly and professionally impossible. Hence, these issues are sufficiently important to be chosen as the topic to initiate this publication.

In the first article, O'Shea and Jessee provide an overview of the ethical, value, and professional conflicts in family systems therapy. They note that the systems' perspective in marriage and family therapy requires a variety of epistomological, conceptual, and technical shifts from traditional individual therapy approaches. These shifts cause systems therapists to be frequently at odds with client family members, nonsystemically oriented colleagues, and the larger social system. This paradigm clash confronts systems therapists with various ethical, value, and professional practice conflicts. Several dilemmas commonly faced by systems therapists are discussed, along with suggested solutions that incorporate the relevant literature and the authors' own evolving professional ethics.

Articles by Taggart and by Seymour present two perspectives on values in family therapy. The thesis of Taggart's article is that the values discussion among family therapists has suffered because of a reluctance to bring values under the same systems epistemology as are other aspects of family therapy theory. The epistemological renewal, currently underway in family therapy, provides the basis for a critique of traditional ways of understanding values. Systemic values are conceived as emerging within processes rather than given a priori; therefore, values and ethics refer to the dynamics of evolving systems, not to the vicissitudes of individual rights. Some preliminary observations are offered about the pragmatics of systemic values.

Seymour examines more practical aspects of the therapist's values and therapeutic style. In his review of the literature, he looks at some specific areas of value concerns that may arise in working with families as well as general value issues. Implications for practitioners are also presented.

The next two articles focus on ethical issues. Kaslow and Steinberg concentrate on the ethical and legal consideration in divorce therapy. Their psycholegal perspective calls for ethical and legal knowledge and for the therapist and lawyer to be cooperative professionals. Morrison, Layton, and Newman examine some of the general ethical concerns in therapy, specifically those in family therapy. They also present a survey of ethical conflicts experienced by various professionals and draw conclusions for family therapists.

Bernstein and Ruback contribute articles on legal issues in family therapy. Both authors advocate familiarity with the basic principles of family law and cooperation between lawyers and therapists. Bernstein reviews legal issues that the family therapist should be sensitive to. His review and suggestions will help readers not to be ignorant of the law. Ruback describes the kinds of legal information that family therapists need. He covers legal process, context of family law, and the role of the therapist in legal proceedings. Both articles direct the reader to sources that provide greater legal detail.

In the final article, Sporakowski analyzes regulation of family therapy. His analysis and comments indicate an inconsistency in regulation and raise several points for thoughtful consideration.

Luciano L'Abate
Volume Editor

1. Ethical, Value, and Professional Conflicts in Systems Therapy

Michael O'Shea*
Department of Psychology
Texas Research Institute of Mental Sciences
Texas Medical Center
Houston, Texas

Edgar Jessee*
Family Systems Program
Institute for Juvenile Research
Chicago, Illinois

---

*Both authors are Doctoral Candidates, Family Psychology Program, Department of Psychology, Georgia State University, Atlanta, Georgia.

The authors wish to thank Luciano L'Abate, Greg Jurkovic, Michael Berger, Robert Brown, David Kearns, and Sadell Sloan for their helpful comments on earlier drafts of this article.

One

THE FAMILY SYSTEMS APPROACH IS A RELATIVELY RECENT BUT radically different orientation to the treatment and prevention of emotional distress. It is a shift away from a linear, cause-effect view of psychological dysfunction toward a framework emphasizing interdependence, information-exchange, and circular feedback mechanisms (Hoffman, 1971; Steinglass, 1978). Although systems therapy in actuality is a collection of minimodels (Steinglass, 1978), symptoms are viewed as actively maintained by the current interpersonal context and as serving a regulating, stabilizing, and communication function in that context. Ideologically, the general systems view incorporates the instinctual and environmental determinism of psychoanalytic and learning theories with the autonomy, personal growth, and goal directedness of the existential-humanistic views of behavior and includes the dynamic interaction of social exchange theories. Practically, the systems approach in therapy strives to balance the needs of individual members with the welfare of the social system as a whole (Hines & Hare-Mustin, 1978). Thus, therapeutic application of the systems approach attempts to change the social context of the symptomatic person to ensure successful and lasting treatment outcome.

Although a systematic perspective promises a net gain in degree and stability of therapeutic change, under certain circumstances this approach is adopted at significant cost to its adherents and participants. On a societal level, systems therapists and their clients may frequently be at odds with other systems and social institutions. American cultural ideology and legal tradition emphasize self-sufficiency, value individual accountability, and sanction individual rights over group preferences. In contrast the systems orientation embodies what Bandura (1978) called "reciprocal determinism," and views the individual as most definable and understandable within a social context of roles and relationships based on mutual constraint/enhancement (Laszlo, Levine, & Milsun, 1974). This clash creates predictable kinds of ethical, value, and professional practice dilemmas for the systems therapist.

To date, these binds have not received sufficient attention in the family therapy literature. In this article, we examine common forms of ethical, value, and legal conflicts facing the systems therapist in his or her professional practice. We argue that these conflicts are concrete manifestations of the philosophical and ideological clash of family systems theory, individually oriented theories of psychological disturbance and treatment, and the social institutions and cultural standards espousing individualism. We do not attempt an exhaustive examination of these conflicts in view of the wide range of preferred assumptions and strategies within family systems therapy (Gurman & Kniskern, 1981b), as well as within individual therapy. We also recognize the gap in any therapy between therapists' theoretical beliefs and their behavior toward particular clients in specific circumstances. Nevertheless, we believe that certain kinds of issues and situations can be problematic to some degree for most therapists who routinely attempt systemic change, notwithstanding the fact that the systems approach shares a code of ethical principles similar to other approaches (AAMFT, 1981). We illustrate some ways in which the adoption of a systems approach, by the nature of this treatment orientation as described earlier, (a) complicates exponentially the kinds of ethical, value, and practical dilemmas that concern therapists of individual orientations and (b) creates a new set of conflicts neither addressed by nor considered relevant to the responsible practice of individual therapy approaches.

CONFLICTS AMONG THERAPIST, COLLEAGUES, AND SYSTEM MEMBERS

When therapy involves two or more persons as clients *and* the therapeutic focus is the current social relationships, there is a quantum increase in the number of possible conflicts and pitfalls that may arise. The systems therapist's professional ethics and values are keyed to enhancing the well-being of the client system. However, this is easier to state in principle than to implement in clinical practice. The myriad of dilemmas stemming from treating the system as the client can be meaningfully subsumed under the following topics, each of which will be discussed in detail: therapeutic use of power, sharing-withholding information (confidentiality), use of paradoxical prescription, tolerating individual members' distress in the service of systemic change (side taking and blaming), and iatrogenic effects (relapse/deterioration) in therapy.

Therapist's Use of Power

Regardless of whether the style of systems therapists is directive or reflective, symptom strategic or growth oriented in approaches to families (what Beavers, 1981, has dubbed "leaping" versus "inching"), there appears to be an evolving consensus among them that a position of power and influence must be established early in treatment (Haley, 1976). Although therapist authority and influence are endorsed in most individually oriented treatment approaches, it is particularly important in working with a family or marital system. The family comes into therapy with a history of day-to-day shared styles of communication and an implicit meaning pattern and relationship rules imbedded in what may appear to an outsider as extraneous, insignificant, conventional behavior (Watzlawick, Beavin, & Jackson, 1967). Therapists are not privy to the special importance of these behaviors within the system, putting them at an initial disadvantage, not unlike that of a new member seeking entry to a secret organization without benefit of the password. The therapist's process of establishing rapport and joining with family members requires deciphering the communications and cracking the code of the family's meaning pattern. This enables the therapist to recognize, intervene, and assign new meaning to, and ultimately change, destructive interactional patterns in the family.

The importance of an active therapist is indicated by studies of negative outcome of systems therapy (Gurman & Kniskern, 1978a). To be effective, a therapist needs to be influential. Early in therapy, systems therapists gain influence with their clients by being active. This way of achieving influence contrasts with their more reflective and insight-oriented individual therapist colleagues, whose influence is conferred by the client's distress and the nature of the therapy contract. Wachtel (1979), commenting on the conceptual and stylistic shifts in moving from individual to family therapy, noted that the reflective stance common in individual therapy is possible largely because the individual therapist's power and influence are products of client distress and transference, as well as therapist skill. She acknowledged her difficulty in being more active while having to share more control over content and direction of sessions with a family, and in feeling less important and central to a client family because of diluted and diffused transference.

A frequent, and often the earliest, test of the therapist's influence in the system arises when the therapist is still an outsider and centers on the issue of who shall attend the sessions. Napier and Whitaker (1973, 1978) have called this the "battle for structure," stressing that the therapist must maintain control over who shall be present in sessions. Napier and Whitaker see the battle for structure as the family's attempt, whether overt or covert, to control the therapy and resist change by dictating the terms of therapy. More often than not, the absent member(s) is symptomatic and is crucial to understanding and dealing with the basic problem. That the therapist must prevail on this issue is crucial to some approaches within the systems view and is consistent with most systems therapy modes. However, value and possible ethical conflicts arise when the therapist, in accordance with Napier and Whitaker's position, decides to refuse or withhold treatment from a family who is resisting in bringing in all members. Particularly for systems therapists in public agencies, such a withholding of services is legally, ethically, and politically questionable, given that such agencies are tax supported, legally mandated to serve those seeking assistance, and often funded on the basis of number of symptomatic clients served.

It could be argued that withholding treatment in the battle for structure does not constitute a refusal to provide mental health services. It is rather an insistence on providing services appropriate to the nature of the difficulty, and thus, it is a responsible, competent, professional practice. An analogy can be made to medical practice in which a physician orders tests and prescribes medications appropriate to the patient's illness or injury and not primarily or solely on the basis of the patient's wishes.* However, psychotherapy in general and family systems therapy in particular do not have medicine's empirically established data base for effectiveness of specific treatments for particular disorders (Gurman & Kniskern, 1981a). Teismann (1980) has faulted the tactic of withholding treatment in the battle for structure on entirely different grounds, namely, that it denies services to motivated family members while risking an implicit alliance between therapist and the resistant member(s). He discussed a variety of strategies for involving unwilling family members short of refusing or withholding services.

---

*This analogy was first suggested to us by Douglas Carl in a personal communication, February 1980.

A frequently adopted solution to the ethical ambiguity and value conflict of withholding treatment in the battle for structure is to offer brief, limited exploratory sessions to the family members willing to come in while advising them that change is not likely to occur or endure unless and until all important members attend. However, this practice and those suggested by Teismann may simply trade one set of ethical/value conflicts for another, since the rationale for attendance of all important members is, with the possible exception of conjoint marital therapy (Gurman & Kniskern, 1978b), a matter more of the therapist's ideology and clinical judgment than of empirically established effective practice. Even if there were a consensus among systems therapists that lasting change depends on the presence of all key family members (which there is not), this position conflicts with the legal right of a person to refuse treatment (Hines & Hare-Mustin, 1978).

An additional ethical implication of the battle for structure was raised by Silber (1976), who noted in discussing individual therapy that regardless of the cumulative data on psychotherapy effectiveness, the consequences of therapy are unpredictable in specific cases, and indeed, not everyone can or should benefit from therapy. This point is even more germane to systems therapy as a relatively recent treatment approach, the effectiveness of which has yet to be empirically documented (Gurman & Kniskern, 1978a, 1978b, 1981a). Thus, it appears that the systems therapist who insists that all family members attend therapy sessions makes a leap of faith, believing that what may be beneficial for the system as a whole will be equally good for individual members. Additionally, such a stance implicitly promises the recalcitrant member's enhanced wellbeing, an outcome that the therapist is not in a position to guarantee (Hare-Mustin, 1980).

Confidentiality and Information Sharing

Confidentiality is closely related to the therapist's use of power and influence and in deciding who must attend therapy sessions. This issue has at least three aspects: information sharing among and between family members, sharing information between the family and outside persons or agencies, and therapist self-disclosure to a client couple or family. The first aspect is more problematic in systems therapy than in individual therapy, since the therapeutic contract is with several people. Haley (1976) has discussed at length the first type of confidentiality, equating the therapist's power and influence in the system with his or her ability to control the flow of information among family members. Haley (1976) emphasized that restricting availability of information creates or maintains boundaries; sharing information weakens or removes boundaries. Haley advised therapists to make it clear to the clients that therapists retain the right to reveal secret information when they deem it appropriate. Haley seems to take a pragmatic, utilitarian position on this issue, defining ethical therapist behavior as whatever is consistent with achieving carefully considered therapeutic goals.

Karpel (1980) discussed the relevant ethical and practical considerations of handling family secrets and confidentiality. He agrees with Haley that knowledge and information bestows power on the knowing person(s). Karpel made a useful and relevant distinction between secrecy and privacy, in terms of how relevant the information is to the unaware member(s). Karpel provided several illustrations. One spouse who does not tell the partner about an extramarital affair maintains a secret, in the sense that mutual trust and reciprocity are violated. Similarly, parents who withhold from a child the fact that the child is adopted violate that child's right to a self-definition and identity that incorporate true genetic/ ethnic heritage. By contrast, Karpel noted that well-resolved traumatic events or previous relationships prior to a parent-child relationship are private rather than secret information. Karpel advocated a therapeutic policy of "accountability with discretion" by which a therapist's decision to share or withhold information is made in terms of the rights and overall well-being of the unaware family member(s). He argues that the therapist who agrees to keep a secret colludes with that person and betrays the trust of the unaware member(s) while enhancing the secret-holding person's power in the family. Such keeping of secrets by the therapist or family members may be a well-intentioned effort to protect family members from possible destructive effects of knowing the secret. Karpel warned, however, that this stance runs the risk that the secret-holding member will unexpectedly reveal the secret information to the others, bringing about the effects feared by the therapist and demolishing the newly aware member's trust in the therapist. Karpel acknowledged that often therapists' need to know (relevant information for assessment and treatment purposes) and their obligation to maintain trustworthiness are in conflict. He offered the preventive solution that the therapist should consult with the family in the initial session regarding how they prefer secret information to be handled.

Less clear-cut are instances in which the therapist finds it necessary to include in therapy significant others who are not nuclear family members, such as friends, neighbors, former spouses, extended family members, or people with whom one or more family members have an antagonistic relationship, such as a former spouse or current lover (Napier & Whitaker, 1978). Such widening of focus challenges conventional ethical guidelines for maintaining confidentiality in individual therapy. Although there is precedent for this notion in the expanded limits of confidentiality maintained in group therapy, the inclusion of a significant "outsider" to assist in evaluation of treatment presents a more ambiguous challenge to customary notions of confidentiality. This person may not share the involvement or investment in therapy outcome that family members presumably have, yet the presence of this person may be needed in some situations to increase commitment of family members to the therapy process and ensure a desirable outcome. However, even with the consent of all family members, including such a significant other person in the sessions takes the risk that this less invested person may subsequently disclose session material to others outside the family. In our view, professional ethics and responsibility require a therapist to first determine that including such people is therapeutically justifiable and is not solely a compensation for the therapist's limited skills and expertise in dealing with systems and particular kinds of problems.

Gumper and Sprenkle (1981) have recently examined the repercussions of current legal definitions of privileged communication in therapy. They concluded that variations and ambiguity in state legal statutes present particularly thorny legal problems and ethical quandaries for system therapists. Specifically, Gumper and Sprenkle noted that ownership of this privilege resides with the client(s), not the therapist. Thus, as these authors observed, a symptomatic client family member in a divorce or child custody proceeding may waive his or her privilege, putting the therapist in the position of having to legally establish that other therapy participants are the therapist's agents in therapy to safeguard their privacy. Potentially more damaging is the fact that many state statutes governing privileged communication in therapy appear to be limited to communications between therapist and client and not to the communications between family members during therapy. Gumper and Sprenkle point out that this appears to sanction one member testifying about another member. It is unclear whether a court would accept the validity of the systems view of the family as an organic unit, particularly in cases in which an extended family member or nonmember was included in the therapy. The authors concluded that the therapist would be ethically and legally well advised, when deeming expanded participation appropriate, to obtain written promises from all participants not to attempt to legally force disclosure of information.

A third aspect of confidentiality and information sharing that is less frequently discussed is the withholding of information, giving of factually false information, or otherwise influencing the client outside of the client's awareness by the therapist. The systems approach lies somewhere between the nondirective analytic therapies that favor an authoritarian, reflective therapist as guardian of the patient's process of insight and self-healing and the directive, confrontative, humanistically-oriented approaches that view the therapy process as a partnership based on mutual self-disclosure between equals. Haley (1976) noted that therapeutic ethics that require therapists to disclose to the client everything they sense about the client are historically recent and falsely assume that therapists are always aware of why they respond in a particular way toward a client. Haley maintained that the problem-oriented therapist functions as a trained expert, not an equal partner with the client. In problem-oriented systems therapy, selective disclosure of observations by the therapist allows the therapist to maintain power and influence in the system and to bring about planned therapeutic change.

Use of Paradox

Selective disclosure by the therapist often involves disclosing factually skewed information to the client couple or family in the form of symptom prescription or other types of paradoxical intervention. Largely through the work of the Mental Research Institute (Watzlawick, Weakland, & Fish, 1974), paradox has become associated with systems therapy. In many reframing or relabeling strategies all therapists, regardless of their orientation, in effect highlight some facts and ignore, deemphasize, or avoid others. Even though such therapist behavior clearly constitutes selective (and as some critics may charge, capricious) distortion of information or facts, the ethical issue involves the question of whether, in so acting, the therapist is deceiving or harming the client. We agree with Fisher, Anderson, and Jones (1981) that when these interventions are effective, they are effective precisely because they are *truthful,* in the sense that they accurately embody each member's phenomenological experience of being involved in a dysfunctional system (Watzlawick et al., 1974).

Such techniques are clearly unethical if they undermine the trust necessary for a therapeutic relationship; if they are used in a kneejerk, cavalier fashion; if they cause the family to feel misunderstood and discounted (Stuart, 1980); or if they mask the therapist's countertransference (Fay, 1976), lack of skill, or faulty diagnosis (Fisher et al., 1981). Ultimately, ethical, responsible use of such techniques requires therapist competence, understanding of the role of the symptom for each family member, adequate supervision/consultation, a therapeutic style conducive to their use, and a sense of proper timing gained through clinical experience (Fisher et al., 1981), as well as a conceptual rationale for choice of type and content of paradoxical intervention (Rohrbaugh, Tennen, Press, & White, 1981; Tennen, Rohrbaugh, Press, & White, 1981).

The common practice of prescribing paradoxical tasks or tasks without an explanation or rationale to the clients raises additional ethical issues, since the therapist can never be certain how a system will absorb and respond to a given intervention (Selvini-Palazzoli, Boscolo, Cecchin, & Prata, 1978). Given the wide range of possible responses, use of these tasks comes close to being based on faith. Even if there is a short-term improvement following adherence to an interactional task, there is no empirical evidence that systems reorganize to maintain the change, or that if they do, the changes generalize to other problematic situations. Gurman (1978) noted that paradoxical reframing and interactional tasks used without explanation or education may at times prolong the system's dependence on the therapist's skill, preventing the system from developing its own coping mechanisms. However, if the intervention is both truthful as discussed earlier and truly systemic (i.e., it includes and affects all members and employs language or metaphor syntonic with members' subjective experience of their family life), the family will more likely identify with the task, change in a more functional manner, and experience the change under its own direction (Selvini-Palazzoli, Boscolo, Cecchin & Prata, 1978).

Limits of Tolerable Distress

The systems therapist's allegiance to fostering need-fulfilling, growth-producing relationships in addition to promoting the autonomy and well-being of individual members casts into sharp relief the ethical-value question pertinent to all therapies: How much short-term distress or risk of harm to the client should be tolerated for the sake of more enduring positive change? The systems therapist who seeks relationship change as primary or equal to intrapsychic change faces a corollary conflict: How much distress or risk to one member should be tolerated for the sake of long-term benefit to the marital relationship or family system? This is a central ethical dilemma if the therapist accepts the notion that the symptomatic member serves a homeostatic, protective, stabilizing function in the family. Clearly, many families who manifest a rigid scapegoating pattern toward one or more members have elected certain members to bear the brunt of systemic discomfort and have in effect made this decision for the therapist. When the therapist attempts to intervene, the symptoms are likely to escalate accordingly. Indeed, to counteract this rigid homeostatic pattern, the therapist may elect to increase individual distress to a crisis level in order to force a fundamental change in the system (Hoffman, 1971).

This ethical conflict has been muted somewhat by more recent trends in family systems theory toward viewing the family system as discontinuously evolving (i.e., characterized by permanent instability, such that symptoms are more accurately "signs of hope" and harbingers of impending developmental transformation; Hoffman, 1981). With respect to value conflicts and cognitive dissonance in the therapist, however, these recent reformulations may only serve to shift the conflict away from therapist-family members to the therapist and his/her nonsystemically oriented colleagues and wider system of mental health helping professionals. The therapist who attempts to precipitate a structural shift in the system by tolerating or deliberately intensifying the distress in the system does so in opposition to the medical ethic and cultural expectation that helping professionals should relieve rather than prolong suffering. Clearly, a physician, despite the use of anesthetics, often inflicts immediate pain on the patient in the process of restoring a more global and long-term health. In systems therapy, however, the distress must at times be amplified before the family is motivated to change its dysfunctional avoidance behavior patterns. The therapist must, as it were, overcome the self-anesthetizing effect of the family's dysfunctional interactions by getting the family to experience the full thrust of anxiety and tension.

Some examples will illustrate this value conflict. One form of paradoxical intervention examined by Fisher et al. (1981) is symptom escalation to a crisis state. This technique is best used to force highly resistant, rigid families to fundamentally alter their dysfunctional patterns of behavior. Fisher et al. cautioned that such a broadside assault on the family rigidity is justified only if less disruptive measures have failed, if the risk of negative outcome is small, and if the current homeostatic pattern is worse than other possible alternatives. However, the therapist is rarely able to precisely predict or control how the system will reshape itself to such an intervention in a crisis and ultimately can do little more than hope for a better outcome.

Particularly difficult for the systems therapist are cases involving physical or sexual abuse of children by adult family members. The common legal and preferred therapeutic response is to protect the victim by removing the abused or abusing member(s) from the family (Anderson & Shafer, 1979). However, the systems therapist who believes that the victim in the family actively fulfills and maintains this role may opt to treat the family while allowing the abused and abusing member(s) to remain in the home for the sake of more stable, enduring (i.e., systemic) change.

When the family presents suicidal behavior as the primary symptom, treatment decisions are even more precarious. The systems therapist faces a trade-off between conservatively safeguarding the suicidal patient through immediate hospitalization, at the cost of reinforcing an active scapegoating process, versus risking self-harm to the suicidal member by avoiding hospitalization in favor of outpatient family treatment (Langsley & Kaplan, 1968). Suicidal persons are usually ambivalent about life and death and function on a continuum of lethality in which the current interpersonal context is salient. The systems practitioner who is prepared to accept increased risk to the suicidal member for the sake of a more favorable long-term outcome must also be prepared for censure by nonsystemically oriented colleagues. It should be noted, however, that including the family system in the evaluation and treatment of a suicidal member may reveal that what may appear as a mild suicidal risk when viewed in isolation can be deemed more serious when seen in the context of a lethal family system (Richman, 1979).

A similar but less dramatic conflict faces the systems therapist who delays or avoids use of drug treatment of proven effectiveness for a severely depressed, manic, or psychotic patient. The therapist may remain loyal to personal values and theoretical position at the cost of negligence or malpractice charges from the client or from nonsystemically oriented colleagues. The implication is not meant to imply that systems therapists never ally themselves with one family member against others and always ignore the symptoms. Rather, as Haley (1976) advised, the therapist must not form a stable alliance with one member against others over the course of the therapy, either by keeping secrets or by overprotection of the scapegoated, symptomatic family member. Yet, as Wachtel (1979) noted, this position (against permanent sidetaking and the systemic view of the symptomatic person as one who actively maintains that role in the family) often conflicts with a common tendency among individual therapists to hold the parents responsible for the client's problems to reduce client guilt and increase self-esteem.

The essential point is not that systems therapists typically avoid special placement, hospitalization, or drug treatment of symptomatic family members out of either personal preference or theoretical persuasion. Rather, it appears that these types of cases often present more acute value conflicts for systems therapists than for therapists of more traditional orientations. In these situations, the therapist must ultimately balance the safety and immediate well-being of individual members with effective systemic treatment considerations (Hines & Hare-Mustin, 1978). The ultimate goal remains a "restoration of balanced reciprocity of fairness" (p. 267) in family relationships (Bosznormenyi-Nagy, 1974).

Equally as controversial as specific techniques are possible risk-benefit contraindications for systems therapy itself. Guttman (1973) reported case histories of four young adult males who showed an increase in suicidal-psychotic symptoms during family therapy. These patients were similar in terms of their marked anxiety, inability to express feelings, and ambivalent, dependent parent-child relationships. Guttman concluded that family therapy initiated soon after a psychotic episode threatened this dependency and triggered the psychotic relapse. Unfortunately, she dwelled more on the vulnerability of the symptomatic child than on the inappropriate use of cathartic or insight-oriented approaches to families in crisis, fueling the suspicion that the "family therapy" employed was more accurately the presence of the family in the treatment of symptomatic individual. The reader could have been better served by a discussion of the relative merits or (in)appropriateness of certain interventions, and the homeostatic function of symptom relapse, than a blanket caveat for all forms of family therapy with recently identified psychotic patients. Bloch and LaPerriere (1973) felt that the only contraindications for family therapy are refusal of the family to be seen as a family (presumably distinguishable from the "battle for structure") and therapist incompetence to work with families. More is known about the negative effects of therapist style than the negative consequences of systems approaches as methods of treatment (Gurman & Kniskern, 1978a).

It could be argued, as Guttman (1973) acknowledged, that the psychotic episodes could have been managed within ongoing family therapy, that they could have been a turning point toward a positive outcome, or that the episodes might have recurred even if family therapy had not been initiated. In any event, the issue of risk-benefits limits is clouded by the fact that depending on the nature of the particular family system, the role of the symptoms as deviation counteracting (Hoffman, 1971), and the therapist's strategy as discussed by Fisher et al. (1981), an initial escalation of symptoms can reflect either a therapist's impotence or his/her considerable (and eventually positive) impact on the family.

Iatrogenic Effects

The amount of risk and distress that a specific family member can bear and should be permitted by the therapist in the service of systemic change raises the problem of negative outcomes in systems therapy. Although the concern for negative effects is shared by practitioners in all treatment approaches and theoretical orientations, systems therapists, like group therapists, must expand their scope of responsibility to include all participants in the therapy. The risk in systems therapy is that a previously asymptomatic family member may become symptomatic during or subsequent to therapy. As Grosser and Paul (1964) noted, this phenomenon is not unique to family therapy, but it is a more salient issue in family therapy because it can be more easily detected and effectively managed in family therapy. Indeed, in certain family systems it can be a positive development for an overly functioning member to become symptomatic (Boszormenyi-Nagy, 1974).

Gurman and Kniskern (1978a) made an important and relevant distinction between relapse and deterioration in therapy. They defined relapse as a negative change occuring between posttreatment and follow-up in the direction of pretreatment level of functioning. Deterioration is viewed as a negative change or escalation of symptoms *during* treatment. Thus, the risk of deterioration poses a more serious and immediate ethical conflict to the therapist than does the risk of relapse, since a relapse at worst indicates that the treatment was ineffective rather than harmful.

Gurman and Kniskern (1981a) recently refined these ideas into policy recommendations regarding design and scope of family therapy outcome research. They advocated outcome assessment at the levels of the identified patient, the marriage, and the family units. They also postulated a hierarchy of positive outcome with minimal acceptable improvement defined as change occurring solely in the symptomatic individual. Optimal benefit is present when improvement extends to the cross-generational relationship level in both the immediate and extended family. By contrast, deterioration is considered to be most harmful when it is confined to the individual and least destructive (and more therapeutically manageable) when it is diffused throughout the system. Gurman and Kniskern's multitiered outcome mapping strategy increases the likelihood that deterioration will be detected when it can be most harmful.

Gurman and Kniskern (1981a) also invoked Parloff's (1976) distinction between mediating and ultimate goals of therapy. Mediating goals are criteria of progress toward the ultimate goals that specify when and how therapy has been successful. They pointed out that deterioration may be a mediating goal in cases in which symptom escalation is necessary for ultimate systemic change. These factors notwithstanding, systems therapists, by virtue of dealing with a client system able to resist change in a myriad of ways, face a more acute, amorphous, and continuous challenge to personal values and therapeutic ethics, compared to their individual therapist counterparts.

THERAPIST-FAMILY-SOCIETAL CONFLICTS

Even though family systems theory approaches symptomatic persons in the context of a dysfunctional family, families are themselves part of a larger social-cultural system. This self-evident fact presents some troublesome ethical and value dilemmas to the systems therapist. Some examples have been recently discussed in the literature. Sonne (1973) has discussed the problem of psychiatric diagnosis for third-party reimbursement and has suggested reliance on adjustment reaction in receiving reimbursement for systems therapy. Hare-Mustin (1980) cited the risk that some systems therapists may subordinate the needs of female family members to the (male-defined) needs of the family by explicitly or implicitly endorsing traditional sex roles and division of labor in the family. The result may be that the personal growth and fulfillment of one or more members (usually females) in nontraditional directions are stifled. Conversely, a therapist can err by encouraging a more contemporary relationship inconsistent with the values of one or more members, such as attempting to equalize the power in a marriage in which one spouse is rigidly dominant and the other rigidly submissive, in accordance with their ethnic values. Stuart (1980) cited a situation in which a wife facing an "empty nest" may be depressed, lonely, and unfulfilled due to cultural or religious sanctions against working women. Direct intervention to increase the wife's independence would lift the depression at the expense of violating the couple's values. A more general pitfall is the therapist's implicit endorsement of an attempt to encourage conformity to the nuclear family structure of the American middle class. A therapist may inappropriately provoke inordinate conflict among family members by fostering autonomy, differentiation, cohesiveness, sobriety, or emotional expressiveness in a form or to an extent that violates the family's racial, socioeconomic, or cultural values (McGoldrick & Pearce, 1981).Often examples include viewing cohabitating multigenerational households, step-families, single parent families, or extended family members living in close proximity as dysfunctional according to white middle-class standards. Clearly, in certain ethnic religious cultures or regions, children remaining at home to care for parents is both sanctioned by the value system and highly adaptive. Although most of these errors are likely due to therapist inexperience, it is clear that the various schools of family systems theory and therapy are not value free (Hines & Hare-Mustin, 1978;Hare-Mustin, 1980).

At a time of declining publicly funded services for the poor and needy, therapists working with such families are likely to grapple more acutely and frequently with the dilemma that encouraging family systems to become more self-reliant may be inconsistent with current economic realities. Self-reliance may be understood by the family or by the larger society as a coded endorsement of or docile compliance with repressive welfare laws and regressive policies favoring curtailment of social service programs. Even though client advocacy and social activism may well be the most productive way to achieve long-term stability in the economically disadvantaged family, we endorse Haley's (1976) view that in the end, the therapist's prime responsibility is to help the client, not to seek institutional change while the client is in distress.

With so many ethical pitfalls and value conflicts the question that arises is, On what basis does a systems therapist decide whether and how to responsibly intervene in a family/marital system? Halleck (1978) held that therapists' knowledge and experience allow them to assess whether intervention might be helpful and how best to proceed to ensure that it will be beneficial. Unfortunately, the present lack of standardized systems therapy training coupled with the plethora of professional allegiances of systems therapists (Group for the Advancement of Psychiatry,

1970) do not ensure that the knowledge and clinical experience of practitioners will always be adequate for this task (Gurman & Kniskern, 1978a). Ultimately, each therapist must be his/her own judge and jury in this matter until uniform certification regulations and ethical standards for systems therapists are adopted and implemented (AAMFT, 1981) and a more solid data base for systems therapy outcome is established (Gurman & Kniskern, 1978b, 1981a).

Ethical therapist behavior clearly requires more than good intentions, and the values permeating therapeutic efforts must, as Abroms (1978) pointed out, be more than a matter of personal bias and subjectivity. Abroms advocated a hierarchy of therapeutic values adopted from Kohlberg's (1969, 1971) scheme of value development, such that therapy is best conducted as a process of "properly staged exposures to ideals" (Abroms, 1978, p. 14), along with an invitation to the client to adopt a more synthesized, comprehensive, and socially integrated value system. If therapeutic ethics involve the determination of what the therapist ought to do to provide maximum benefit for the greatest number of people, then systems therapy as a treatment of social relationships would seem to be the most ethical and integrated of therapies. Yet, as has been illustrated, systems therapy as a treatment of social relationships is also subject to the widest range of possible ethical conflicts and value clashes, as well as a host of administrative dilemmas addressed elsewhere (Framo, 1976, 1978; Haley, 1975).

CONCLUSION

Wahlroos (1976) observed that family therapy, like any new approach that grows out of the limitations of existing therapies, initially tended to overstate its position and range of appropriate use. The systems practitioners have been preoccupied with staking out and defending their turf and rather self-righteously differentiating themselves from their predecessors. Only recently have they focused sustained attention on the ethical aspects of the systems therapy enterprise. This article has discussed and illustrated how ethical issues, therapist, family and societal values, codes of professional conduct and legal issues overlap and merge in everyday clinical practice to present a variety of problematic situations. Certainly the conflicts caused by the meshing of ethical issues, societal values, codes of professional conduct, and legal issues can be avoided or minimized if careful attention is given to informed consent, therapeutic contracting, and specification of policies and procedures (Hare-Mustin,

Marecek, Kaplan, & Liss-Levinson, 1979; Stuart, 1980). However, to the extent that the problems discussed stem from a paradigm or epistomology clash between the systems approach and individually oriented therapy approaches and legal traditions, these conflicts will continue to confront the systems therapist in a variety of forms. They merit continued consideration and discussion by systems therapists.

REFERENCES

Abroms, G.M. The place of values in psychotherapy. *Journal of Marriage and Family Counseling*, 1978, *4*, 3-17.

American Association of Marriage and Family Therapists, New AAMFT code of ethics adopted. *AAMFT Newsletter*, 1981, *12*, 1-3.

Anderson, L.M., & Shafer, G. The character-disordered family: A community-treatment model for family sexual abuse. *American Journal of Orthopsychiatry*, 1979, *49*, 436-445.

Bandura, A. The self system in reciprocal determinism. *American Psychologist*, 1978, *33*, 344-358.

Beavers, W.R. I don't know. Why don't you agree with me? *AAMFT Newsletter*, 1981, *12*, 3-4.

Bloch, D.A., & LaPerriere, K. Techniques of family therapy: A conceptual frame. In D.A. Bloch (Ed.), *Techniques of family psychotherapy: A primer*. New York: Grune & Stratton, 1973.

Boszormenyi-Nagy, I. Ethical and practical implications of intergenerational family therapy. *Psychotherapy and Psychosomatics*, 1974, *24*, 261-268.

Fay, A. Clinical notes on paradoxical therapy. *Psychotherapy: Theory, Research and Practice*, 1976, *13*, 118-122.

Fisher, L., Anderson, A., & Jones, J.E. Types of paradoxical interventions and indications/contraindications for use in clinical practice. *Family Process*, 1981, *20*, 25-35.

Framo, J.L. Chronical of a struggle to establish a family unit within a community mental health center. In P.J. Guerin, Jr. (Ed.), *Family therapy: Theory and practice*. New York: Gardner Press, 1976.

Framo, J. L. Personal reflections of a family therapist. *Journal of Marriage and Family Counseling*, 1978, *4*, 15-28.

Grosser, G., & Paul, N. Ethical issues in family group therapy. *American Journal of Orthopsychiatry*, 1964, *34*, 875-884.

Group for the Advancement of Psychiatry. *Treatment of families in conflict: The clinical study of family process*. New York: Aronson, 1970.

Gumper, L. L., & Sprenkle, D. H. Privileged communication in therapy: Special problems for the family and couples therapist. *Family Process*, 1981, *20*, 11-23.

Gurman, A. S. Contemporary marital therapies: A critique and comparative analysis of psychoanalytic, behavioral and systems theory approaches. In T. J. Paolino & B. S. McCrady (Eds.), *Marriage and marital therapy: Psychoanalytic, behavioral and systems theory perspectives*. New York: Brunner/Mazel, 1978.

Gurman, A. S., & Kniskern, D. P. Deterioration in marital and family therapy: Empirical, clinical and conceptual issues. *Family Process*, 1978, *17*, 3-20. (a)

Gurman, A. S., & Kniskern, D. P. Research on marital and family therapy: Progress, perspective and prospect. In S. L. Garfield & A. E. Bergin (Eds.), *Handbook of psychotherapy and behavior change* (2nd ed.). New York: Wiley, 1978. (b)

Gurman, A. S., & Kniskern, D. P. Family therapy outcome research: Knowns and unknowns. In A. S. Gurman & D. P. Kniskern (Eds.), *Handbook of family therapy*. New York: Brunner/Mazel, 1981. (a)

Gurman, A. S., & Kniskern, D. P. (Eds.), *Handbook of family therapy*. New York: Brunner/Mazel, 1981. (b)

Guttman, H. A. A contraindication for family therapy. *Archives of General Psychiatry*, 1973, *29*, 352-355.

Haley, J. Why a mental health clinic should avoid family therapy. *Journal of Marriage and Family Counseling*, 1975, *1*, 3-13.

Haley, J. *Problem-solving therapy: New strategies for effective family therapy*. San Francisco: Jossey-Bass, 1976.

Halleck, S. L. *Treatment of emotional disorders*. New York: Aronson, 1978.

Hare-Mustin, R. T. Family therapy may be dangerous for your health. *Professional Psychology*, 1980, *11*, 935-938.

Hare-Mustin, R. T., Marecek, J., Kaplan, A. G., & Liss-Levinson, N. Rights of clients, responsibilities of therapists. *American Psychologist*, 1979, *34*, 3-16.

Hines, P. M., & Hare-Mustin, R. T. Ethical concerns in family therapy. *Professional Psychology*, 1978, *9*, 165-171.

Hoffman, L. Deviation amplifying processes in natural groups. In J. Haley (Ed.), *Changing families: A family therapy reader*. New York: Grune & Stratton, 1971.

Hoffman, L. Behind the looking glass: A bicameral model for therapy. *AAMFT Newsletter*, 1981, *12*, 3, 8-10.

Karpel, M. A. Family secrets: I. Conceptual and ethical issues in the relational context: II. Ethical and practical considerations in therapeutic management. *Family Process*, 1980, *19*, 295-306.

Kohlberg, L. Stage and sequence: The cognitive developmental approach to socialization. In D. A. Goslin (Ed.), *Handbook of socialization theory and research*. New York: Rand McNally, 1969.

Kohlberg, L. From is to ought. In T. Mischel (Ed.), *Cognitive development and epistomology*. New York: Academic Press, 1971.

Langsley, D. G., & Kaplan, D. M. *The treatment of families in crisis*. New York: Grune & Stratton, 1968.

Laszlo, C. A., Levine, M. D., & Milsun, J. H. A general system framework for social systems. *Behavioral Science*, 1974, *19*, 79-92.

McGoldrick, M., & Pearce, J. K. Family therapy with Irish-Americans. *Family Process*, 1981, *20*, 223-241.

Napier, A. Y., & Whitaker, C. Problems of the beginning family therapist. In D. A. Block (Ed.), *Techniques of family psychotherapy: A primer*. New York: Grune & Stratton, 1973.

Napier, A. Y., & Whitaker, C. *The family crucible*. New York: Harper & Row, 1978.

Parloff, M. B. The narcissism of small differences—and some big ones. *International Journal of Group Psychotherapy*, 1976, *26*, 311-319.

Richman, J. Family therapy of attempted suicide. *Family Process*, 1979, *18*, 131-142.

Rohrbaugh, M., Tennen, H., Press, S., & White, L. Compliance, defiance, and therapeutic paradox: Guidelines for strategic use of paradoxical interventions. *American Journal of Orthopsychiatry*, 1981, *5*, 454-467.

Selvini-Palazzoli, N., Boscolo, L., Cecchin, G., & Prata, G. *Paradox and counterparadox*. New York: Aronson, 1978.

Silber, D. E. Ethical relativity and professional psychology. *Clinical Psychologist*, 1976, *29*, 3-5.

Sonne, J. C. Insurance and family therapy, *Family Process*, 1973, *12*, 399-414.

Steinglass, P. The conceptualization of marriage from a systems theory perspective. In T. J. Paolino, Jr., & B. S. McGrady (Eds.), *Marriage and marital therapy: Psychoanalytic, behavioral and systems theory perspectives*. New York: Brunner/Mazel, 1978.

Stuart, R. B. *Helping couples change, a social learning approach to marital therapy*. New York: Guilford Press, 1980.

Teismann, M. W. Convening strategies in family therapy. *Family Process*, 1980, *19*, 393-400.

Tennen, H., Rohrbaugh, M., Press, S., & White, L. Reactance theory and therapeutic paradox: A compliance-defiance mode. *Psychotherapy: Theory, Research and Practice*, 1981, *18*, 14-22.

Wachtel, E. F. Learning family therapy: The dilemmas of an individual therapist. *Journal of Contemporary Psychotherapy*, 1979, *10* (2), 122-135.

Wahlroos, S. Some limitations of family therapy. *Journal of Family Counseling*, 1976, *4*, 8-11.

Watzlawick, P., Beavin, J. H., & Jackson, D. D. *Pragmatics of human communications: A study of interactional patterns, pathologies and paradoxes*. New York: Norton, 1967.

Watzlawick, P., Weakland, J. H., & Fish, R. *Change: Principles of problem formation and problem resolution*. New York: Norton, 1974.

2. Linear Versus Systemic Values:
Implications for Family Therapy

Morris Taggart, Ph.D.
Houston-Galveston Family Institute
Houston, Texas

Two

IT IS A DELICIOUS IRONY THAT TOWARD THE END OF A decade in which the development and proliferation of *clinical techniques* emerged as a major fascination in family therapy (the 1970s), there should also be a revival of interest in epistemology and related topics (Colapinto, 1979; Dell, 1980, 1981a, 1981b; Dell & Goolishian, 1979; Elkaim, 1981; Keeney, 1979; Keeney & Sprenkle, in press). This epistemological renewal promises to challenge the fondest concept and most cherished technique in family therapy. The area of values is not exempt.

It is the thesis of this article that the values discussion among family therapists has suffered because of a reluctance to bring values under the same systems epistemology as informs other aspects of their work. The fulfilling of systems theory, implicit in the epistemological renewal, provides a context for an exploration of values that takes the system seriously.

THE EPISTEMOLOGICAL RENEWAL

Family therapy may be viewed as a "research program" (Brown, 1977) that came into being because existing research programs in psychotherapy failed to find adequate solutions to their own problems. No matter how previous research programs seemed to differ from each other, they all developed in the context of an already developed view of reality. The advent of family therapy, in effect, was a turning away from this customary epistemology. Instead of relegating "family" to what happened in the gaps between the substantial attributes of isolated entities, the new model viewed the family as a "system in process."

But all research programs run into problems, that is, if they are any good. For one thing, it is unlikely that all of the richness implicit in a paradigmatic shift would be grasped immediately. A rediscovery of seminal contributors like Bateson (Dell, 1980; Dell & Goolishian, 1979; Keeney & Sprenkle, in press) has meant that the existing presuppositions of family therapists are as apt to be questioned as any other (Dell, 1981b). Again, the idea of a paradigmatic shift does not imply that all who made the leap into the new way of thinking landed in the same neighborhood. They did not jump off from the same place; hence, they define the place differently. That the diversity of family therapy, mapped so dramatically by the *Handbook of family therapy* (Gurman & Kniskern, 1981), extends to the epistemological level as surely as to the levels of theory and technique is not an unreasonable assumption. The assumptions that permit an observer to punctuate a pattern into aggregates judged to be similar allow for the punctuation of the same pattern at the finest level of specificity. A more specific classification (punctuation) system will yield less similarity. Ultimately, and always, epistemologies are personal.

The development, then, of family therapy has been such that there can be no established once-and-for-all body of knowledge that can only be developed like Catholic dogma. What we have instead is a homologue of the "primeval soup" (Miller & Orgel, 1973)—a rich mixture of epistemologies, theories, clinical techniques, professional groupings, friendship/enemy networks, and much more besides—in which almost anything can happen and probably will.

The willingness to "go back to the origin," whether it be the contributions of seminal thinkers like Bateson (1972, 1979) or simply questioning one's deepest assumptions, has the effect of creating "the possibility of recognizing and bringing into play . . . new development lines" (Jantsch, 1980, p. 300). One of these "new development lines" is a new openness to what is happening in other branches of human activity. Family therapy, after all, is but one aspect of a broader restructuring of human thought, underway in a general sense for the past half-century. Jantsch (1980) has called this "the metafluctuation which rocked the world" (p. 8) and insists that it extends to all human endeavor. Some aspects, indeed, of this shift in paradigm, such as the ecology movement and holistic medicine, may have penetrated further into the public consciousness than has family therapy. In the circumstances following the oil boycott of 1973, deeply held notions about the meaning of national sovereignty came under severe challenge. Multinational trading blocks (e.g., the European Economic Community) and multinational companies are major expressions of the process that seeks to transcend static national boundaries.

It is, however, in the turmoil called *modern science* that most farreaching effects of the restructuring may be seen. Even a cursory view of 20th century science makes it clear that established results are the least established aspect. The only permanent aspect of science is the process of research (Brown, 1977), and it is the consensual operation of the scientific community that guarantees validity, not indubitable findings or indubitable methodologies. Reductionism and separatism are transcended as discoveries in one field set up reverberations in others. Major breakthroughs such as identification of the background radiation and the discovery of black holes in space have heralded an unprecedented widening of the scope of human observation of the total cosmic system. As when the family therapist widens the angle of observation by bringing other family members into the process, these developments have led to a new appreciation of the dynamic connectedness of all things within a universe which is unfolding openly but coherently (Jantsch, 1980).

The insistence that the pattern of connectedness is dynamically unfolding, rather than structurally based, is at the heart of the matter. For more than 2,000 years, Western science has been devoted to a recognition of structure—the "building blocks" of matter—in an attempt to reduce the whole into its parts. Earlier forms of systems theory tended to continue this tradition through a commitment to such structural notions as homeostasis and adaptation (Dell & Goolishian, 1979). Such emphasis on steady-state dynamics proved to be of inestimable value in technology, especially in the control of complex machinery. By contrast, however, no living system can ever be permanently stabilized. The dynamics of living systems prescribe no output beyond self-organization and self-renewal. The order through fluctuation principle announced by Prigogine and his collaborators (Nicolis & Prigogine, 1971, 1977; Prigogine, 1976) is revealed in open systems that are far from equilibrium. Under the older, static view, increasing complexity inevitably leads to instability (May, 1973). Self-organizing, nonequilibrium systems may, however, be unstable, yet they may survive by evolving new structures. These new structures are not permanently stable but *metastable;* that is, a system *itself* structures its existence in space and time so that its own dynamics might unfold. Metastability is, then, delayed evolution (Jantsch, 1980, p. 255). The higher the resistance against structural change, the more powerful the fluctuations that will break through eventually. Thus, metastability implies both the destruction of the old structures and the push into equally temporarily stabilized new ones. Such notions about how systems maintain order *through* change are, of course, already being applied to the pragmatics of family therapy (Elkaim, 1981).

But dynamic connectedness points to what might be the most radical step of all—the idea that the dualism of mind and nature no longer serves humanity well and the assertion that it must be overcome. The more traditional view of the evolution of mind, indeed of life itself, has left people of the Western world with a profound sense of separateness from all that is. Now the evolution of mind (and humanity) is seen as taking place according to the same processes as have brought other aspects of the cosmos to its present pattern. Jantsch argues that all aspects of human evolution, whether biological, sociobiological, or sociocultural, are connected through *homologous* rather than *analogous* principles, that is, principles which have common origins rather than mere formal similarity (Jantsch, 1980). Thus, the development of life (mind) is not an event that happens *in* the universe or *over against* it. Nor is mind any longer seen as that exclusive attribute of humankind by which it contemplates the cosmos. Said nondualistically, mind activity is inseparable from the matter in whose dynamics it expresses itself. That is what Bateson meant when he equated mind with the cybernetic system (Bateson, 1979). No longer, then, do we think of humans as evolving in a static environment. Evolution proceeds on both the macroscopic and microscopic levels, and both are aspects of the same unified and unifying evolution. Evolution no longer applies only to a vertical dimension—a coherence in time—but also a horizontal dimension—a coherence in space. Family-of-origin theory has emphasized coherence within the time dimension (time-binding), especially as this is punctuated by the appearance of separate generations. Strategic theory, on the other hand, appears to operate within the coherence found in horizontal relationships in the present (space-binding). A truly comprehensive family theory will surely have to take account of both aspects of evolutionary process and especially *the interactions between them.*

If, as argued here, humanity and all its activities (including the development of family therapy theories) are clearly within evolutionary process, the most human question is to ask if it has a special place. Most answers draw distinctions between the human species and nature. Thus, humanity is seen as higher on the evolutionary ladder as compared with other life forms or subsystems. Rather than speak of a special place for humankind (e.g., in structural terms such as status or right), it is more fruitful to talk about our function as that part of the process that has entered fully into co-evolution with itself and, because of its connectedness *to* all that is, *with* all that is. We perhaps live simultaneously at more levels than other subsystems. As our consciousness of the various levels on which we live expands (i.e., as the sense of connectedness is heightened and broadened), the rules and theories by which we impose order on the patterns of life change.

Humanity may be on the brink of taking its place within nature, but not if it leaves the deepest aspects of life, meaning and values, outside. If the new epistemology makes it difficult to see an individual family member as the site of pathology, it may make it equally difficult for family therapists to proceed in the values domain in the traditional way.

LINEAR VALUES AND THE EPISTEMOLOGICAL CHALLENGE

The premises of Western epistemology, particularly those that promote a profound disinterest in connectedness and process, virtually insist that values be seen as originating outside the system. Humanity-as-ego (Watts, 1961, p. 173) is alienated from its organic life, from other human beings, and from the cosmos in which it lives. It is hardly surprising that we should seek the meaning of life outside the system as well. Thus, ethics in Western philosophy tend to be understood in metaphysical terms, and consequently, as being valid in some absolute sense (Jantsch, 1980, p. 263). As Jantsch notes, the only legitimate response to values originating outside the system is adaptation.

Dell (1981a) reminds us that time is not considered to be a fundamental aspect of reality in Aristotelian epistemology. Logic is not "within time" nor, according to Plato, are Beauty, Truth, or Virtue. Indeed,

> *Plato thought nature but a spume that plays*
> *Upon a ghostly paradigm of things*
> —Yeats (1928)

Thus, the eternal verities float somewhere above or behind this shadowy vale of tears in contextless purity, uncontaminated by the dross of what actually happens. Once again, adaptation seems the only proper posture.

A modern variant of this position is the view that social change is permitted only within the restraints of unchanging social values, and that the institutions that support and promulgate these unchanging values must themselves survive without change (Jantsch, 1980).

In short, traditional ethics and ways of dealing with values exhibit a view of reality that is marked by a structural rather than a process orientation, homeostasis and adaptation rather than order through fluctuation, and the need for "unmoved movers" (Dell, 1981a) as a guarantee of universal and eternal validity. Small wonder, then, that Western ethics has developed rules for behavior that are primarily interested in promoting the welfare and development of individuals (Jantsch, 1980, p. 265). After all, a process that led to a thorough exploration of the possibilities of atomism, separatism, and reductionism within and between the other disciplines can hardly be supposed to have exempted the field of values. So, when insurance companies defend their refusal to reimburse policyholders for family therapy as a *matter of ethics,* it might make sense to take them seriously.

Nowhere is Western philosophy's focus on the individual more apparent than in the worldwide concern for rights of one sort or another. Hare-Mustin (1978, 1980; Hines & Hare-Mustin, 1978) has brought that concern into the family therapist's office. Perturbed by the risks she discerns as inherent in giving priority to the good of the family-as-a-whole over individual members' rights, she has listed particularly the right not to be treated, the right to confidentiality, the right to privacy (not to be embarrassed, exposed, etc.), and women's rights in the area of power. But raising questions about rights—understood as inalienable, individual, and axiomatically supreme—at the logical level of family or system may be no more than the same epistemological error which insists that a family member's "schizophrenia" be treated as an entity distinct from the family's pattern. If the family is an aggregate of individuals with respect to rights, why not for personality structures as well? This view is consistent with Hare-Mustin's statement that "some family members have successfully *disengaged* themselves from an 'enmeshed' family . . . so requiring them to become *involved again* (through participation in family therapy) is not in their best interests" (1980, p. 935, italics added). Disengaged is but one in an ecology of positions taken by members of an enmeshed family, and the judgment that one position is better than another might be hard to sustain. An emotional cutoff (Carter & McGoldrick Orfanides,

1976) does not end emotional processes within and between family members; in fact, it intensifies them. That, of course, might be helpful but hardly in the context of a rights paradigm that is characterized by a linear, structure-oriented, defensive point of view (Vickers, 1973).

Others within family therapy have discussed the values aspects of their work. Some (Grosser & Paul, 1971; Haley, 1976) have restricted their inquiry to professional ethics, others (Duhl & Duhl, 1981) to making their values assumptions explicit, whereas perhaps only one major theory (Bosznormenyi-Nagy & Spark, 1973; Bosznormenyi-Nagy & Ulrich, 1981) has included the values dimension as a basic aspect. These contributions have not excited any great response from the field and, with the possible exception of Bosznormenyi-Nagy, are not considered by many to be the salient contributions of these writers to family therapy theory.

How to understand the relative silence on the topic of values among family therapists is not clear. It is not, perhaps, an unreasonable assumption that family therapists also have assumed that values are given in some way quite distinct from how other aspects of theory are developed and, in consequence, feel little need for values to be brought under the same systems epistemology. The fulfilling of that systems epistemology may, however, provide the basis for new initiatives in the values area.

SYSTEMIC APPROACHES TO VALUES

The proposal thus far is an insistence that theories, paradigms, and ways of "doing" values, themselves unfold according to the rules of the game of evolutionary process. Paradigms do not accumulate knowledge in the way that equilibrium structures (e.g., crystals) grow; they evolve through instability phases to new metastable structures (Jantsch, 1980, p. 290). The instability derives not only from the falsification of the old structure (as research programs succeed in exposing their limits) but also from the openness of the dynamic regime represented by the paradigm. The emerging new structures, at most, take over subsystems of the old structure without change. More likely, however, these old concepts are retained with changed meanings (Brown, 1977, p. 167). What has been referred to here as the epistemological renewal is an instability phase in the unfolding of family therapy, though not confined to it. This renewal, and others yet to come, will challenge the deepest assumptions of family therapists about what we think we know and how we know it.

The unity of mind and nature, so important an emphasis of the new epistemology, places the human species, mind, and values squarely within an evolutionary framework. Values and ethics now refer to the dynamics of evolving systems and not to the vicissitudes of individual rights. Thus, Churchman (1968) calls for the study of "the ethics of whole systems" in which he assumes that "sector ethics" and "system ethics" are usually at variance. Jantsch (1980) considers that many values, traditionally associated exclusively with humans, have in fact emerged much earlier in evolution. Thus, the value of error correction appears at the level of the gene; the value of variety, at the level of ecosystems; flexibility in coping with the unexpected, at the level of multi-cellular organisms; and so on. Emergent *human* ethics, in which morality is a manifestation of multilevel consciousness, *enhances* evolution, and in some sense *is* evolution, in that it operates at the highest levels of dynamic connectedness. Evolutionary ethics, therefore, not only transcend the individual but, as is the case in ecological planning, all of humankind as well, that is, if mind and nature are truly one.

The multilevel aspect of systemic values presents something of a difficulty to traditional ethics because of the latter's tendency to operate serially on single levels. If declining stocks of fossil fuels are bad, then the invention of the electric car will be hailed as good. If, on the other hand, the cost (economic and ecological) of tremendously increased demands for electricity are added, the bargain may not be as appealing. An argument could be made, surely, for the hope that current efforts to develop an electric car will fail. Only then, perhaps, will society tackle the problem of how to move around crowded cities without having to pay homage to everyone's inalienable right to private transportation in urban areas. A multilevel approach robs one of the facility with which distinctions between opposites are customarily made. By contrast, the rights paradigm is committed to a *distinction of opposites* that is restricted in practice to "bargaining in small steps." Rather than enhancing evolution, such ways of dealing with values result in stabilization and rigidification of existing structures. As noted earlier, of course, such delayed evolution merely paves the way for even greater fluctuations to break through eventually. Nor is one way of getting to the point of dealing with the fluctuation (e.g., declining stocks of fossil fuels) just as good as any other. The way a thing happens *is* the thing, and some ways of approaching the crisis may be more creative (less destructive) than others. This is what is involved in Jantsch's notion of *gliding evolution* (as over against *quantum jumps*) in which the interplay of many small changes replaces radical restructuring of the system (Jantsch, 1980). The recent trend to more fuel-efficient automobiles, first among foreign manufacturers and later in the U.S. domestic market, is hopefully an example of gliding evolution. Planning undertaken with system-sensitive values in view enables a system to develop new metastable structures, some of which might be transitional in the short run, which avoid or ameliorate the disruptions associated with quantum jumps. The development of family therapy as a way of assisting families, not so much to avoid change as to make it less destructive, is based on the same premise.

Inherent in any discussion about change is the issue of continuity/discontinuity (Dell & Goolishian, 1979). When, as described earlier, a system enters an instability phase, the perturbation that drives the system across the threshold of stability into a new regime is determined by stochastic (random) processes. Not only is it impossible to predict which fluctuation will be crucial, but it is impossible to describe in advance the new metastable structures that emerge as a consequence. This is discontinuous change. At the same time, however, there is a loose use of the term *discontinuous,* which tends to suggest that the new structures are *totally* discontinuous with previous manifestations of that system. This is a view that is perhaps more characteristic of those who emphasize pragmatics over aesthetics (Keeney & Sprenkle, in press). A theorist who emphasizes space binding over time binding (e.g., a strategic therapist) is more likely to describe change as discontinuous. There are two objections to excess in this direction. First, from an epistemological point of view, discontinuous appears to mean little more than unexpected as defined by an observer. It is the observer's map (theory, paradigm) that supplies the apparent discontinuity. In observing discontinuous change, an observer is learning more about the system as it presents itself, and the map is called into question. Second, systems theory points to the dynamic connectedness of all that is. Whatever unexpected changes occur in a system, that system is connected homologously with all systems. If such is the case, why sound trumpets about the system's discontinuity with its previous manifestations? Too large claims about discontinuity, especially in relation to a therapist's interventions, may have to do with the *hubris* of therapists who want to make their work more special than it is.

Similar error is courted when second-order change is distinguished radically from first-order change in a way which suggests that one is more real or better than the other. Just as "music is about silence" (Brendel, 1981), each concept needs the other for its own explication and operation. Thus, it is not unusual for strategic therapists to underline how many previous and unsuccessful attempts at therapy their clients have experienced before coming for the real thing. What is missing is any acknowledgment that those other experiences in any way contribute to what the strategic therapist-and-client system is able to accomplish.

The question of continuity/discontinuity takes on peculiar poignance in the values discussion. Values to some are the *only* things that last, and to tamper with the method embedded in those *lasting values* is to risk being accused of overturning them. Systems, however, are organized as to operate in some sort of balance between confirmation and novelty (von Weizsacker & von Weizsacker, 1974). Total confirmation would refer to a system in thermodynamic equilibrium, which, for living systems, equals death. Total novelty, on the other hand, refers to a system in chaos, which, in living systems, heralds disintegration. Life, as always, is lived in the dance between. Watts (1961) uses language as a metaphor for the tension between confirmation and novelty (continuity and discontinuity). A language that is all innovation runs the risk of losing its coherence. A language that has stopped growing is in danger of becoming a relic. Any proposal to approach values differently unfolds within the context of the old values, ensuring both debate and a common task.

But, it still may be asked, does not this emphasis on evolutionary ethics, which emerge with and within evolutionary process, destroy the possibility of ethics, since it removes responsibility from the individual person? Does not all this talk about systems leave a diminished role for the individual—perhaps no role at all? Questions about the role of the individual in the context of family therapy are being raised (Duhl & Duhl, 1981; Gurman, 1980; Taggart, 1981), and even as thoroughgoing a systems thinker as Minuchin (1979) has wondered if family therapists have not "gone too close to the other pole, sometimes approaching the human being as a mere respondent to field forces" (p. 6). Williamson (1981) makes a great deal of the concept of *personal authority* and ponders its destruction by an excess of systems thinking. However, it is precisely at this point where evolutionary theory has anticipated these questions and, perhaps, shows the way. Humanity is not the product of evolution—it is its human expression. Indeed, the role of fluctuations renders the law of large numbers invalid and gives a chance to the individual and its creative imagination. The concept of co-evolution includes that of co-responsibility. In the sociocultural phase of evolution, the individual becomes co-responsible for macroevolution. Thus, when a person is engaged, say, in a process of differentiating oneself from within the family, that person is the family in evolution! Thus, evolutionary creativity—the thoughts, feelings, ideas, plans, visions—is not directed *against* evolution, but rather represents a new development line in which the family, community, society, and civilization become more of what they are. As evolutionary process focuses more and more on the individual, it acts in such a way as can only be described as "elitist" (Jantsch, 1980, p. 270).

Another way of making the same point is to say that the direction of evolution is toward complexity, novelty, and creativity. Bateson (1972) noted that evolution proceeds from the "adjusters" (animals that adjust their body temperature to that of the environment), through the "regulators" (that maintain constant body temperature), to the "extraregulators" (humans who create their own environment in the form of heated and cooled shelters). The earlier life forms were by far the best adapted, but human beings have far more freedom in deciding where to live.

Perhaps, then, it is time for a new focus on the individual within the system. There is the danger, of course, that any attempt to avoid an "upward reductionism corresponding to a purely spiritual life which remains without consequences" (Jantsch, 1980, p. 259) will fall into a downward reductionism of "unmoved movers" (Dell, 1981b) and linear notions of power (Keeney, 1979). It is one thing to chide the anthropomorphism implicit in saying that "systems experience" (Duhl & Duhl, 1981). It is quite another to notice the *anthropocentrism* in saying that "only individual human beings experience."

THE PRAGMATICS OF SYSTEMIC VALUES

Having pointed out family therapy's relative failure to bring values under the constraints *and* the opportunities of systems thinking, pragmatics at the level of a code of behavior is hardly possible. Nonetheless, the pragmatics of systemic values is an essential ingredient in its unfolding. This is doubly true for clinicians, especially those interested in epistemology. It is seeing and using what one knows to be so (order through fluctuation, self-reference, multilevel reality, etc.) that saves one from resenting clients as intrusions. It also saves clients from having to sit through long lectures on "the positive value of fluctuations." Thus, however, tentatively, some preliminary observations about the pragmatics of systemic values are offered.

Example

The family consisted of father, mother, and 16-year-old son, with two older young adult members away at college. The family's distress was centered on the 16-year-old's struggle to get a family-purchased new car 2 years before his high school graduation—the point at which his siblings had received theirs. An early impression of the therapist was that the father was cast in the role of defender of the family's explicit value system; the son was Anarchy herself bent on destroying those values; and the mother played the part of double agent to both sides.

Discussion

At the outset, the father clearly wanted to deal with the issue at the level of son's rebellious/maybe mentally ill nature. This is the minimum loop of the practical person (Churchman, 1968) who decides what the problem is and moves to eliminate it. The son, well trained by this time, wanted to do likewise, except that it was the father's unreasonableness/ meanness that was now the problem. The mother, tired of chauffering her son to a multitude of activities but convinced of the value of values, teetered and tottered between support for her husband and financing the revolution.

Starting as early as requiring all three protagonists to come in together, the ensuing process saw the problem go through a number of transformations that enlarged the family's awareness of the contexts in which it manifested itself. Thus, the single-level approach of individual attributes (values) was soon abandoned for a multilevel one that included levels such as the relation between father and son, the basic triangle among parents and son, the older children's feelings and ideas about the problem, how neighborhood families dealt with the matter of cars and high school students, the extended family's practice with cousins the same age as son, the family's economic condition, the father's feelings about his job, and so on. In the face of absurd comments from the therapist on whether or not car manufacturers were losing sleep nights awaiting the outcome, the family took to the polling of friends and relatives as eminently sensible. Somewhere around the eighth session, the father was 20 minutes late in coming to the weekly meeting. He had been talking to a friend at work who had a *used* car for sale and, if the son were willing to take a look at it the following week-end . . . . The rest was easy.

Even as bloodless a description as the one just stated is of a process that twisted and turned in all sorts of directions; the deliberate choice of the therapist to pursue a multilevel reality brought other aspects of systemic values to view. The canvassing of friends and relatives was an example of space-binding, as was the discussion of the family's economics. A conversation about how much things had changed since the parents were teenagers points to time-binding. Every move to a new level was experienced as a disruption (nonequilibrium). The major effect, perhaps, was the new sense that family members (those who attended sessions and those who did not) had of actively participating in creating the emerging design of the family's life (co-evolution and co-responsibility). Family values were no longer defined as father's (or son's, or mother's, or the therapist's) values writ large, but represented a new dimension that emerged within the process. Even the crucial intervention of the father's co-worker is instructive. If a therapist is accustomed to highlighting those *therapist interventions* that *change* the family's operations, he or she may feel cheated in not being in at the kill. If, on the other hand, a therapist is tuned-in to the connectedness of all that happens, including events punctuated as outside the therapy, such linear notions of cause and effect vanish.

Thus, the evolutionary paradigm is not restricted to the development of family theory (systemic values) in general, but now refers to the unfolding of a particular process involving a specific therapist with an actual family. How the therapist views values is an important link between these two levels of operations. This, in turn, brings the discussion back to where it began—the question of the therapist's epistemology. The central question of the pragmatics of systemic values is now revealed. Which paradigm informs the therapist's own unfolding with respect to values?

CONCLUSION

Family therapy has achieved much in its short history. In concert with systems thinkers in other disciplines, family therapists have translated a major fluctuation in human thought into a pragmatic regime that affects the daily lives of countless people. In doing so, family therapists have contributed much to the fluctuation, from the arcane reaches of epistemology to the recruitment of trainees intrigued with tuning-in to the fluctuation. A field that has survived nonexistence, subsequently to emerge as a scandal, a fad, one modality among many, and finally a minor bandwagon, now faces the greatest danger of all—its own success. The appurtenances of having arrived—professional associations, degree programs, journals, model *curricula,* codes of ethics, licenses, third-party payments, and government-stamped accreditation programs—all point to the fact that if much has been gained, much can be lost. Can the continued unfolding of family therapy survive the *metastable* structures that are a part of that unfolding? But, then, this is *always* the question. The dance is one, the beat goes on.

REFERENCES

Bateson, G. *Steps to an ecology of the mind.* New York: Ballantine, 1972.

Bateson, G. *Mind and nature: A necessary unity.* New York: Bantam Books, 1979.

Boszormenyi-Nagy, I., Spark, G. *Invisible loyalties: Reciprocity in inter-generational family therapy.* New York: Harper & Row, 1973.

Boszormenyi-Nagy, I., & Ulrich, D. N. Contextual family therapy. In A. S. Gurman & D. P. Kniskern (Eds.), *Handbook of family therapy.* New York: Brunner/Mazel, 1981.

Brendel, A. *Dick Cavett show.* Public Broadcast System, May 26, 1981, KUHT T.V., Houston.

Brown, H. I. *Perception, theory and commitment.* Chicago: University of Chicago Press, 1977.

Carter, E. A., & McGoldrick Orfanides, M. Family therapy with one person and the therapist's own family. In P. J. Guerin (Ed.), *Family therapy: Theory and practice.* New York: Gardner, 1976.

Churchman, C. W. *Challenge to reason.* New York: McGraw-Hill, 1968.

Colapinto, J. The relative value of empirical evidence. *Family Process,* 1979, *18,* 427-441.

Dell, P. F. The Hopi family therapist and the Aristotelian parents. *Journal of Marital and Family Therapy,* 1980, *6,* 123-130.

Dell, P. F. Paradox redux. *Journal of Marital and Family Therapy,* 1981, *7,* 127-134. (a)

Dell. P. F. Some irreverent thoughts on paradox. *Family Process,* 1981, *20,* 37-42. (b)

Dell, P. F., & Goolishian, H. A. Order through fluctuation: An evolutionary epistemology for human systems. Paper presented at the Annual Scientific Meeting of the A. K. Rice Institute, Houston, Texas, March 1979.

Duhl, B. S., & Duhl, F. J. Integrative family therapy. In A. S. Gurman & D. P. Kniskern (Eds.), *Handbook of family therapy.* New York: Brunner/Mazel, 1981.

Elkaim, M. Non-equilibrium, change and change in family therapy. *Journal of Marital and Family Therapy,* 1981, *1,* 291-297.

Grosser, G. H., & Paul, N. L. Ethical issues in family group therapy. In J. Haley (Ed.), *Changing families: A family therapy reader.* New York: Grune & Stratton, 1971.

Gurman, A. S. Behavioral marriage therapy in the 1980s: The challenge of integration. *American Journal of Family Therapy,* 1980, *8,* 86-96.

Gurman, A. S., & Kniskern, D. P. (Eds.). *Handbook of family therapy.* New York: Brunner/Mazel, 1981.

Haley, J. *Problem-solving therapy: New strategies for effective family therapy.* San Francisco: Jossey-Bass, 1976.

Hare-Mustin, R. T. A feminist approach to family therapy. *Family Process,* 1978, *17,* 181-194.

Hare-Mustin, R. T. Family therapy may be dangerous for your health. *Professional Psychology,* 1980, *11,* 935-938.

Hines, P. M., & Hare-Mustin, R. T. Ethical concerns in family therapy. *Professional Psychology,* 1978, *9,* 165-171.

Jantsch, E. *The self-organizing universe: Scientific and human implications of the emerging paradigm of evolution.* New York: Pergamon Press, 1980.

Keeney, B. P. Ecosystemic epistemology: An alternative paradigm for diagnosis. *Family Process,* 1979, *18,* 117-129.

Keeney, B. P., & Sprenkle, D. H. Ecosystemic epistemology: Critical implications for the aesthetics and pragmatics of family therapy. *Family Process,* in press.

May, R. M. *Stability and complexity in model ecosystems.* Princeton, N.J.: Princeton University Press, 1973.

Miller, S. S., & Orgel, L. E. *The origins of life on earth.* Englewood Cliffs, N.J.: Prentice-Hall, 1973.

Minuchin, S. Constructing a therapeutic reality. In E. Kaufman & P. N. Kaufmann (Eds.), *Family therapy of drug and alcohol abuse.* New York: Gardner Press, 1979.

Nicolis, G., & Prigogine, I. Fluctuations in non-equilibrium systems. *Proceedings of the National Academy of Science,* 1971, *68,* 2102-2107.

Nicolis, G., & Prigogine, I. *Self-organization in nonequilibrium systems: From dissipative structures to order through fluctuations.* New York: Wiley-Interscience, 1977.

Prigogine, I. Order through fluctuation: Self-organization and social system. In E. Jantsch & C. H. Waddington (Eds.), *Evolution and consciousness: Human systems in transition.* Reading, Mass.: Addison-Wesley, 1976.

Taggart, M. Abstracts. *Journal of Marital and Family Therapy,* 1981, *7,* 96.

Vickers, G. *Making institutions work.* London: Associated Business Programmes, 1973.

von Weizsacker, E., & von Weizsacker, C. *Offene systeme I: Beitrage zur zeitstruktur von information, entropie und evolution.* Stuttgart: Klett, 1974.

Watts, A. *Psychotherapy east and west.* New York: Random House, 1961.

Williamson, D. S. Personal authority via termination of the intergenerational hierarchical boundary: A "new" stage in the family life cycle. *Journal of Marital and Family Therapy,* 1981, *7,* 441-452.

Yeats, W. B. Among school children (poem). In W. B. Yeats (Ed.), *The tower.* New York: Macmillan, 1928.

3. Counselor/Therapist Values and Therapeutic Style

Warren R. Seymour, Ph.D.
Department of Educational and Counseling Psychology
University of Missouri-Columbia
Columbia, Missouri

Three

"BE NOT LIKE THE LAME SELLING CRUTCHES; AND THE blind, mirrors" warned Gibran (1923). This admonition could well be applied to the values held by counselors and therapists and their proper place in the therapeutic process. We must be aware of, admit to, and try to understand fully the impact of personal values as we go about our day-to-day business of marriage and family counseling. If we are indeed, even occasionally, selling our values in one form or another to our clients, we should at least be aware of what it is we are selling, and, the consumer client should rightfully demand from us "truth in packaging."

Hammer (1972), commenting on the current state of the art in psychotherapy, declared that from the available research, it is clear that the primary determinant, as far as therapeutic effectiveness was concerned, is the therapist. Positive therapeutic change by the client, added Hammer, is not related to any particular kind of school, technique, or theory of psychotherapy. If such is the case, and I believe that it is, then the values held by counselors, along with their other personal characteristics, must also be related to therapeutic effectiveness. Such personal characteristics and the way that an individual counselor integrates them into the counseling process represent that counselor's therapeutic style, for better or worse.

No two clients are exactly alike. Certainly no two couples or families are identical. In a profession that demands great tolerance of ambiguity from its practitioners, there are few constants to cling to in the helping professions. The counselor's therapeutic style is one variable that is present in all therapeutic interactions and, therefore, does represent a constant of sorts. In referring to counseling style as a variable, however, it is implied that even though it is always present, it is not always constant as the counselor behaves, interacts with, and relates to the client. Nor would we want it to be so. Nonetheless, it behooves us to try to understand the counselor variable and the effect that it may have on the process and the outcomes of counseling.

Despite the fact that the counseling literature has tended to focus more on client variables than on those of counselors, there has been a considerable research effort to examine the personal characteristics of counselors and how these characteristics relate, if at all, to counselor style and counselor effectiveness. More than 30 years ago, Polmantier (1947) observed that a primary problem in the training of counselors was recruiting counselor trainees with personal characteristics essential to success as a counselor. Almost 20 years later, in a review of the literature on the personality characteristics of counseling students (Polmantier, 1966), he concluded that the same selection problem existed and should be a major concern for the counseling profession. Bost (1970) concurred, stressing the need for more detailed studies of the professional member of the counseling relationship. According to Bost, what happens to the counselor during the counseling process is just as important as what happens to those people the counselor undertakes to assist. "It seems apparent," added Bost, "that the counselor can no longer be ignored" (p. 121).

One such personal characteristic of the counselor that has come under considerable scrutiny over the years is the system of values held by the counselor. A value, as defined by Rokeach (1973), is "an enduring belief that a specific mode of conduct or end-state of existence is personally and socially preferable to an opposite or converse mode of conduct or end-state of existence" (p. 5). Hinsie and Campbell (1970) define a value as "that which is esteemed, prized, or deemed worthwhile and desirable by a person or a culture" (p. 802). Let us take a look at what the literature has to say about counselor values.

COUNSELOR/THERAPIST VALUES

Values in counseling have intrigued researchers for a long time. The focus, however, has been on client values, the values of society, the values of the profession, and the values inherent in the definition of a counselor. Much less is known about the values of counselors as individuals and the impact that these values have on the style and the performance of the counselor. As Hultman (1976) pointed out: "Although a rich body of theory and research deals directly with the complex role of values in human functioning, the implications of this work for counselors and other helping professionals have not been adequately studied" (p. 269). Gass (1970) agreed that the values of the helping person and their effect on the therapeutic process represent a variable that was often unrecognized and rarely discussed.

Maddock (1972) talked about an individual's values as the individual's way of seeing reality. Values are, said Maddock, "the lenses through which he [the individual] views the world as he seeks to achieve self-fulfillment. An individual is emotionally invested in his values so that they become to him unshakably right and therefore he acts in accordance with what he believes" (p. 272). Such a statement has obvious implications for counselors. We do become emotionally invested in our values, we do hold some of them to be unquestionably right, and we do act in counseling in accordance with what we believe. We, as counselors, must be aware of the emotional investment, admit to, and hopefully question those values that have been previously unquestioned, and then examine closely how what we believe influences how we act as counselors. If our values are, in fact, the lenses through which we view the world, then we need to have our vision checked as a part of the selection and training process, and at regular intervals thereafter.

According to Middleton (1970), there is a considerable interaction effect in counselors' development between their cognitive processes and their value systems. The particular conceptual and therapeutic model that any given counselor chooses to use is a result of these forces. Middleton concluded that the value system(s) of counselors can be demonstrated in their results. Gass (1970), reacting to Middleton's article, made an even stronger statement insisting that a therapist should "be acutely aware and sensitive to his own value system whether or not he is of the school that believes in verbal expression of the therapist's feelings" (p. 344). Gass argued that if indeed therapists were not aware of their own feelings, it would be most difficult for them to truly understand the value system of the client.

Hulnick (1977), in an article appropriately entitled "Counselor: Know Thyself," contended that counselors need to resolve value issues for themselves before they can help clients who are struggling with value concerns. In a similar vein, Piel (1979) concurred with an earlier statement by Bergantino (1978) that a lack of self-awareness on the part of the counselor is a "fatal flaw" in counseling. Such self-awareness must extend beyond the recognition of transient emotional reactions and attitudes to an understanding of why we choose to do what we do as counselors.

Every person, in some fashion, struggles with the question of what life is all about. Smith and Peterson (1977b) offered the opinion that such a struggle cannot be successfully resolved with the creation and incorporation of a personal system of values. Translating this belief into implications for counselor/therapist training programs, they stressed the need for more attention to the exploration and clarification of values for such trainees. Smith and Peterson (1977b) affirmed the belief that "until trainees have come to grips with the values that can be expected to appear sooner or later in sessions with their clients, it is to be questioned whether they have been sufficiently prepared" (p. 230). In their view, a values-clarification module should be an integral part of any counselor-training program.

Gutsch (1968) agreed that both the client and the counselor are influenced by the standards of the society in which they exist, and, although the values of the counselor may appear to be independent of those standards, the counselor's inner attitudes will find some expression in the counseling relationship. Smith and Peterson (1977a) reached a similar conclusion: "All that we say and do both as persons and as helpers implies value judgments" (p. 309). Counseling is one means by which individuals examine their values. Such a process should begin by counselors becoming fully aware of their personal values so that they will be less likely to impose those values on their clients. Hudson (1967) put it more forcefully, concluding that the further growth of the profession hinges on the effectiveness with which we, as marriage counselors, can deal with value issues.

In a current book dealing with human values, Kalish and Collier (1981), in discussing psychotherapy as a means of intervention, commented: "Almost nothing that we do is totally free of implicit and explicit values" (p. 246). For that reason, even though some might contend that psychotherapy is value free, they contend that such is not the case. As they put it: "Whether by intent or accident, commission or omission, psychotherapy does not operate in a value-free way" (p. 247). They suggested, as an interesting example of how values might operate in psychotherapy, that "a psychotherapist who would have treated Van Gogh would have implied that it was worth risking the loss of the artistic enjoyment of the rest of the world to save the man's emotional well-being" (p. 246). The implication of what should have been done by the therapist in this example is, of course, a value judgment on the part of Kalish and Collier.

In summary, it seems apparent that there is a lack of solid research in the area of counselor/therapist values, especially research directly related to the family therapist. The whole area of counselor/therapist values is frequently unrecognized, or, if recognized, ignored. The one clear area of agreement in the literature is that values need to be examined as an essential part of the training process for family therapists. The research that is available makes it obvious that values and value issues are closely tied to the results one may expect to achieve as a family therapist.

VALUES AND THE FAMILY THERAPIST

General Value Issues

After introducing the area of therapist values, it is important to examine some general value issues and their relationship to marital/family therapy. Marsh and Humphrey (1953) were among the early writers to speak to this issue: "Cultural tradition molds sex roles and marital difficulties and, for that matter, marital counseling" (p. 32). They warned marriage counselors not to impose the standards of middle-class conventionality upon their clients and proposed that the success of marriage counseling would be in terms of how well counselors addressed the cultural traditions of their clients. What ought to be in a marriage or family has not been adequately defined. Individual therapists should not attempt to impose their definition on unwitting clients.

Value issues in marriage counseling were examined by Hudson (1967). He saw marriage counselors as products of their culture and reflecting personal values in counseling, whether or not the counselors were aware of it. Marriage counselors must be cognizant of their values and how they operate in the course of therapy. Hudson predicted that "if the marriage counselor risks revealing himself from behind the professional shroud of the passive, reflecting, nonjudgmental mummy, it is inevitable that he will express his values, attitudes, and opinions on a wide variety of subjects" (p. 169). Hudson expressed the belief that the very nature of counseling implies a value system. One of the best methods for examining personal values as a counselor is to carefully question the assumptions that are made to support clinical diagnoses. He succinctly summarized: "Psychological jargon and diagnostic categories are all too frequently rationalizations for more fundamental personal values on the part of the counselor" (p. 175).

Kalafat, Boroto, and France (1979), after investigating the hypothesis that counseling effectiveness is at least partially due to the similarity in style and values between counselor and client, concluded that a complex relationship did, in fact, exist among performance, values, and experience level. The use of "self" by a family therapist was examined by Keith (1974). He postulated that family therapists can actually free up members of rigid narrow family systems when they introduce their own affect into the family structure. We can only hope that when they do this they are fully aware of what they are introducing and have, at least, some idea of the potential impact that such affect will produce.

In their analysis of marital role ideals in distressed and nondistressed couples, Frank, Anderson, and Rubenstein (1980) discussed such ideals, or values, in terms of clients only. Nothing was said about how such ideals affect the counselor and, in turn, the therapy. Frank et al. did, however, state as an implication for treatment that it was crucial for the therapist not to assume that traditional marital roles were necessarily satisfying or dissatisfying to either or both members of the couple.

In an article dealing with the defensive projections of values, feelings, and impulses in marriage counseling, Sunbury (1980) examined this behavior on the part of the counselor as well as the client. Sunbury stressed the need for self-awareness and understanding of the nature of such projections so that the counselor can avoid these hazards and view the interactions of the couple more clearly. Leslie (1979) concerned himself with the collective and personal biases of family life education, but much of what he reported could apply equally well to family therapists. After examining such value-laden topics as open marriage, group marriage, living together, no-fault divorce, and dual-career marriages, Leslie concluded that family life specialists have an obligation to ensure that their own advocacy of certain life styles does not induce those with whom they work to choose life styles without full information about them and the alternatives that are available.

Tsoi-Hoshmand (1976) investigated the implications of feminist and humanistic values for marriage and marriage therapy. She bemoaned the fact that so little has been done to conceptualize clearly, or describe in functional terms, the implications of changing values on the reality of spousehood and marital therapy. In her view, the orientation of marital therapists is a function of their own values. Silverman (1973) also reported on the psychological and philosophical implications of value issues in marriage counseling. According to Silverman, marital counseling, as a profession, and counselors, as individuals, need a sound set of values. He goes on to make a case for traditional values in marriage and views marriage as the "core institutional arrangement that binds people together, it is the basic fabric of social structure" (p. 109). This statement, and others in this article, seem to be loaded with the author's own values as to the values that a marital therapist should hold dear.

In a rare example of taking the counselor variable into consideration and going beyond such things as counselor skill and experience level, Neubeck (1973) discussed the process involved in the marriage counseling triad. Neubeck asked, "Does it matter to us if the counselor is a persuader or reflector, shaper or cajoler, listener or manipulator, toucher or distancer . . . " (p. 121). It is the counselor's very participation in the triad that is seen as the instrument of change.

A basic supposition often made by therapists, according to Gass (1970), is that the methodology of therapy will, in some way, reduce to a minimum the imposition of therapist values on the client. Gass (1970) refuted such wishful thinking and posed the question, "If, in the most uncontaminated atmosphere one can create, there is mounting evidence that the therapist's values play a part, how much more are such values playing a role in current variations of clinical techniques and procedures" (p. 343). Gutsch and Rosenblatt (1973), in an attempt to apply a touch of Martin Buber's philosophy to counselor education, studied married couples who found themselves in value struggles that had been intensified due to a lack of dialogue. Counselors in training were seen as particularly vulnerable to the same dialogue blockage because they cling to the mechanics of the relationship, rather than seek the genuineness that such a relationship can bring. When both counselor and clients are experiencing such a blockage, the problems involved in dealing with value struggles are greatly magnified.

Hultman (1976) noted that some counselors only took note of client values when they were at variance with their own values. Clients sensing this may deliberately embrace the values of the counselor to avoid being confronted by the counselor. Responding to the question of how values should be taught, Arcus (1980) made the suggestion that learning to reason about values is the answer. She defined value reasoning as learning to distinguish factual claims from value judgments and learning to clarify one's value sentences. Value clarification for marital enrichment was looked at by Piercy and Schultz (1978). They asked the same question of marital enrichment leaders that I would ask of marital/family therapists in general: "Can therapists or enrichment leaders help couples clarify their values when their own values are not clear or, if clear, assumed to be the right ones for other couples?" Smith and Peterson (1977a) presented an interesting discussion of trends in the handling of values by counselors. They cited the growing recognition that value neutrality on the part of the counselor is an impossibility. As a consequence of this inability to maintain neutrality, counselors must be aware of the values they espouse.

As part of an overview of the field of marriage counseling, Nichols (1973) examined the areas of values and ethics. In his assessment, marriage counseling, at that time, was experiencing considerable strain as the result of value divergencies and differences in outlook among its practitioners. Some of the causes suggested for such divergencies included changing attitudes and increased openness toward human sexuality, changing forms and alternate styles of marriage and family living, changing attitudes toward divorce and remarriage, and a variety of other changes in morals and mores.

Counseling outcomes and their relationship to counselor values would seem to be the "bottom line," as far as the whole area of counselor/therapist values is concerned. Yet, relatively few studies deal directly with this topic. Most outcome studies, such as one by Gurman (1973), focus on other variables such as treatment type, time in therapy, and the effectiveness of single versus cotherapists. Studies of therapist characteristics include variables such as empathic ability and experience, but they seldom examine therapist values and their impact on therapy. Rice, Fey, and Kepecs (1972), for example, looked at therapist experience and style as factors in therapy. They concluded that experienced and inexperienced therapists did have different personal therapeutic styles and that subjectively rated effectiveness was related to therapist "comfortableness." One cannot help but wonder what therapist values were inherent in their so-called personal style and perceived comfortableness. It would appear that few researchers, especially in the family therapy area, are paying attention to Tsoi-Hoshmand (1976), who made the recommendation that "in evaluating relative outcome of different therapy approaches, researchers should take into consideration such value choices" (p. 51).

Specific Value Issues

Family therapy concerns itself with problems and issues that are value-laden and complicated by the fact that many of the values involved are in a constant state of flux. The list is almost endless but would certainly be highlighted by such value issues as divorce, dual careers, birth control, sexual dysfunction, abortion, child rearing, and child and spouse abuse, to name a few. Because such issues are so loaded with values for both clients and therapists, those of us who work in the area of family therapy need to give them more than token recognition. They are not the kind of issues that will allow even the pretense of being value-free when therapists attempt to deal with them. Many of these issues have been addressed in the literature. The questions raised are many, but the answers provided are few.

Sexism

In discussing a feminist approach to family therapy, Hare-Mustin (1978) declared that "the unquestioned reinforcement of stereotyped sex roles takes place in much of family therapy" (p. 181). She suggested that only by becoming aware of their own values and biases could therapists change such sexist patterns. Such biases affect therapist style in many ways, from their style of communicating with their clients to their relabeling deviance in terms of diagnostic labels such as passive-aggressive, phobic, dependent, and so on. Because of value biases, Hare-Mustin raised the question of whether a male therapist can or should work with a female client. It was suggested that therapeutic alliances are often formed between male therapists and male clients because they hold similar value biases. Obviously, such alliances could also be formed between female therapists and their female clients. Tsoi-Hoshmand (1976) advocated that counselors and therapists follow feminist or humanistic values so that marital interventions could move from role-oriented to person-oriented and from open-ended quid pro quos to value-based negotiations. In their discussion of sexist values in the treatment of sexual dysfunctions, Peterson and Peterson (1973) stressed the need for men to better understand the values of women in the area of sexuality and vice versa. Sex-role stereotyping among counselors in training was examined by Burlin and Pearson (1978). They commented on the fact that although sex-role values and beliefs of counselors have been surveyed, little is actually known about the effects that such values have on counselor behavior or style.

They concluded that "for all the speculation about the high level of sex role stereotyping attitudes among persons in the helping professions, there is virtually no research that explores the relationship between these attitudes and helper's functioning" (p. 221). Taking a somewhat different perspective in looking at value issues of concern to feminists, Eisenbud (1977), while examining potential value conflicts between women therapists and women patients, warned that "even when the patient elects a conservative, unliberated alternative, rather than an assertive, revolutionary stance, the female therapist must honor her choice, since there is validity in human interdependence, object love, and procreation needs" (p. 16). Such a warning could well be directed to some male therapists, who have consciously or unconsciously adopted feminist values as the "right" values for the woman of today.

An excellent overview of research findings concerning values, attitudes, biases, and stereotypes held by counselors of women is provided by Nutt (1979).

Sexuality

Values related to problems in the area of human sexuality and the rapid changes in societal values that have occurred in this area have been studied by many researchers. Gordon (1976) commented that the best kind of sex education takes place in the context of responsible values and decision making. The same principle applies when sex education takes place in a private session with a therapist. Kremer, Zimpfer, and Wiggers (1975) examined the values of counselors as they related to homosexuality. They advocated that counselors working with adolescent males should carefully consider their own views about homosexuality and the homosexual activities of their clients if they are to be truly effective. They proposed that "whatever ethical and theoretical position a counselor takes, the counselor must be able to discuss a client's homosexual behavior and the client's feelings about it in a direct, nonthreatening, and open manner, lest a youth's fear, guilt, and difficulty are compounded by the counselor's own fear and indirectness" (p. 99). Thompson and Fishburn (1977) studied the attitudes of graduate counseling students toward homosexuality. They concluded that the students in their study were relatively well informed about homosexuality and had largely rejected most of the common myths and fallacies about homosexuality. Some of the implications for counselor training that resulted from this study are closely tied to the values that counselors have regarding homosexuality. If counselors have unresolved homosexual or homophobic reactions of their own, their counseling effectiveness will be reduced. Counselors need to be comfortable enough with this problem to allow their clients to be homosexual. The counselor should make the client aware of his/her sexual creed so that the client can make an informed decision about continuing therapy. If the client does continue therapy, it is the counselor's responsibility to monitor his/her own values, attitudes, and beliefs to ensure that they do not interfere with the counseling process.

In an attempt to set up guidelines for counseling young people with sexual concerns, Kirkpatrick (1975) stressed the tremendous impact of the rapid changes that have recently occurred in sexual attitudes and behaviors. Such rapid changes make it imperative for counselors to constantly be aware of their own sexuality and their sexual values. Counselors need to be comfortable with their own sexuality before attempting to work with the sexual concerns of others. In the area of sexuality, counselors must learn to display openness, dispassion, and candor. They must separate, as much as possible, their own sexual values from their roles as counselors. As a final suggestion, Kirkpatrick warned that "the counselor should not attempt to convince the client of a viewpoint, no matter how sound the counselor's own reasons for believing that particular point of view" (p. 148).

Melton (1968) also addressed the impact on the marriage counselor who finds himself/herself in the middle of changing sexual values in our society. Such counselors suffer from "value schizophrenia," according to Melton. Counselors must become aware of what their own sexual values are. The sexual values of counselors may be changing just as rapidly as those of their clients. The question becomes, How effectively can counselors function when they are struggling with their own contradictory sexual values while attempting to assist a family faced with a variety of sexual value conflicts? In a cleverly written and imaginative article that attempted to look ahead to sexual value changes, Myers (1973) projected this issue ahead to the year 2020. Sexual values change, but the need for family therapists to come to grips with their own sexual values, as they impact on their therapeutic efforts, remains the same. Roman, Charles, and Karasu (1978) provided an interesting review of the effects of changing sexual attitudes and life styles on the value systems of therapists.

In a study of values related to premarital sex, Lewis and Walsh (1980) compared counselor reactions to explicit versus implicit communication of sexual values and investigated the effects of subject-counselor value similarity on the subject's perception of, and confidence in, the counselor. They found no significant differences in perceptions, but subjects were more willing to see a counselor with values about premarital sex that were more similar to their own. In another investigation of attitudes toward premarital sex, Walker, Somerfeld, and Robinson (1978) surveyed college students' reactions to the psychological and social implications of one-night stands. Over 50% of their sample saw the implications as being negative. Despite the fact that a rather large proportion must not have seen one-night stands as having negative implications, there is little quarrel with the need for family therapists to be aware of current attitudes toward premarital sex if they are to work effectively with family members participating in such activity.

Dual Careers

Dual-career marriages and their implications for therapists were studied by Price-Bonham and Murphy (1980). They saw dual-career marriages/families as high-stress groups presenting unusual challenges for the therapist. Values held by persons in such a marriage/family and those of the therapist working with them are seen as equally important. The therapist must have a clear understanding of his/her own level of comfort and acceptance of such marriages. If the therapist does not, it will be sensed by the clients. Counselor biases should be acknowledged directly. Price-Bonham and Murphy concluded that "the interaction of values of clients and clinicians is a crucial parameter for the clinician's attention. Values are a basic issue with other issues often deriving from them" (p. 186).

Abortion and Sterilization

Abortion and sterilization have been investigated in relation to the values of counselors and their impact on clients wrestling with problems and decision making in these areas. Clark, Bean, Swicegood, and Ansbacher (1979) studied couples who were trying to decide whether the male or the female should undergo sterilization. They emphasized that this was a value area for the couple involved and for the counselor attempting to assist couples in this dilemma. Another study dealing with sterilization (Cole & Bryon, 1973) completely omitted any discussion of values related to sterilization, especially the values of therapists working with couples who were contemplating sterilization. Wright (1972) discussed the psychological aspects of vasectomy counseling. As part of counseling a client who is considering a vasectomy, Wright suggested that "as the counselor encourages the client to reflect on his decision, he also encourages him to evaluate his motivation and expectations more realistically" (p. 265). It would have been helpful if the author had added, "and hopefully do this in an atmosphere free from the counselor's values and biases regarding vasectomies."

Brashear (1973) examined the area of abortion counseling. She pointed out that such clients may be experiencing considerable alienation and other psychological reactions to this crisis, thus making the client particularly vulnerable to the biases of the counselor. Many abortion counselors may find themselves in a personal value dilemma between their client's decision and what they would have chosen. Because of this, not all counselors can or should do abortion counseling. Family therapists need to be aware of their limitations in this area, and, if they cannot resolve their own value conflicts, refer abortion clients to someone who can work with them in an unbiased fashion.

Minorities

Value conflict resolution training for counselors of minority clients was studied by Minor and Minor (1978). They concluded that counselors with cultural and racial values different from those of their clients tended to encounter value conflicts in their attempts to assist such clients. Lager and Zwerling (1980) examined time orientation in relation to therapeutic efforts with ghetto clients. They highlighted the marked contrast between the "present-time cultural value orientation" of ghetto residents' concerns with immediate, real, and psychological survival and the middle-class orientation of most therapists, whose values are oriented toward the future (e.g., the Protestant ethic). As a result, many middle-class therapists misinterpret certain client behaviors as expressions of impulse rather than of culturally determined expectations.

Religion

The religious values of clinicians were the focus of an investigation by Bergin (1980). In his view, the religious values of clinicians are often quite discrepant from the religious values of their clients. He concluded that religious values must be sincerely and conceptually integrated by clinicians if they are to be effective professionals.

Death and Dying

Social values related to death and dying were investigated by Kalish (1972). He contended that practitioners should take great caution before projecting their own values and needs on the dying, especially the elderly. The therapist should support the individual's choice of actions to be taken, rather than those of the well-meaning therapist. Gibbs and Achterberg-Lawliss (1978) discussed the implications of spiritual values in counseling terminal cancer patients. They concluded that counselors must be able to separate their own feelings and values from those of the terminal patient. They stressed that counselors must be able to accurately perceive, and then accept, the patient's value system as being correct for the patient.

Disabilities

Counseling individuals with disabilities is another area fraught with potential value conflicts for the therapist. Nathanson (1979) urges counselors to "become aware of their feelings and thoughts, and to monitor their interactions with disabled clients so that existing beliefs and biases will not interfere with positive client growth" (p. 236). Such beliefs and biases are often deeply rooted and can have a significant effect on the therapy that takes place. According to Nathanson, the effects of such beliefs and biases tend to occur independent of the training, skill, and objectivity possessed by the counselor. His admonition sounds all too familiar: "Counselors must be aware of their own attitudes and consequent behaviors if they are to work effectively with the disabled client" (p. 233).

Because of the paucity of outcome research related to therapist values, most of what has been reported in the literature about the impact of values on therapist behaviors or style has been philosophical in nature, or, in many cases, pure speculation. Although the research is lacking, there is a large literature testifying to the importance of values. The specific value issues discussed previously cover some but not all of such issues that find their way into a family therapy session. Yet, any, or all, could be present within a given family that therapists are attempting to help with a problem that, on the surface, seems not directly related to any of these issues. It is complicated when different members of a family have divergent values about the problem situation. Family therapists must be especially sensitive in detecting their presence and possess a high level of self-awareness of their own values if they are to successfully weave their way through a veritable mine field of values, any of which could figuratively, if not literally, blow up in their face.

IMPLICATIONS FOR FAMILY THERAPY

The proceeding review of the literature reveals that there is good consensus on several points that directly relate to the values of family therapists and their therapeutic style.

- Therapists do have values.
- These values cannot be kept out of the therapeutic process.
- Because therapists' values and value judgments do find their way into the therapeutic process, it is essential that therapists become aware of their values and the impact of those values on their therapeutic style and consequent therapeutic effectiveness.
- Therapist values, and their implications for therapy, are particularly important in family therapy because family issues are characteristically value-laden and often in a state of flux for both the therapist and the various family members.
- Therapist values do influence overall therapeutic style.
- The therapist variable is a crucial, if not the most crucial, determinant of therapeutic effectiveness.
- Since therapist values do influence therapeutic style, they must also influence therapeutic effectiveness.
- Little is known from data-based research about what the actual effects of therapist values are on therapeutic style and effectiveness.

If one accepts the notion that the points listed here do, in fact, have validity for the field of family therapy, then some obvious implications for practitioners of family therapy would certainly include:

- a need for increased self-awareness of our personal values and a concern for the impact that they have on therapy;
- a need for values clarification as a part of the training of family therapists;
- a need for family therapists to continually monitor their personal values throughout their professional careers; and
- a need for more data-based research on (a) the family therapist as a variable in therapy, (b) the relationship of the therapist variable to therapeutic style and effectiveness, and (c) the potential for matching clients and therapist on the basis of their values.

Therapists, especially those in training, do tend to suffer from what Melton (1968) described as value schizophrenia. Value schizophrenia is the split or dichotomy that therapists often experience between the values they actually have and those values that they think they should have as a result of their perception of the ideal family therapist role. Many therapists carry this affliction with them long after they complete their training. It is seldom diagnosed after that point and, therefore, seldom treated. Thus, it is especially important in the training of family therapists to ensure that proper treatment for this malady is initiated as a crucial part of the training program. It is equally important that professional therapists become aware of their values and integrate these values appropriately into their therapeutic behaviors or style.

REFERENCES

Arcus, M. E. Value reasoning: An approach to value education. *Family Relations*, 1980, *29*, 163-171.

Bergantino, L. A. A theory of imperfection. *Counselor Education and Supervision*, 1978, *17*, 286-292.

Bergin, A. E. Psychotherapy and religious values. *Journal of Consulting and Clinical Psychology*, 1980, *48*, 95-105.

Bost, D. L. Changes in altruistic orientations and theory preferences of beginning counselors. *Counselor Education and Supervision*, 1970, *9*, 116-121.

Brashear, D. B. Abortion counseling. *Family Coordinator*, 1973, *22*, 429-435.

Burlin, F., & Pearson, R. Counselor-in-training response to a male and female client: An analogue study. *Counselor Education and Supervision*, 1978, *17*, 213-221.

Clark, M. P., Bean, F. D., Swicegood, G., & Ansbacher, R. The decision for male versus female sterilization. *Family Coordinator*, 1979, *28*, 250-254.

Cole, S. G., & Bryon, D. A review of information relevant to vasectomy counselors. *Family Coordinator*, 1973, *22*, 215-221.

Eisenbud, R. Counter-transference issues in women therapists: Value conflict between women therapists and women patients. *Clinical Psychologist*, 1977, *30*, 14-17.

Frank, E., Anderson, C., & Rubenstein, D. Marital role ideals and perceptions of marital role behavior in distressed and non-distressed couples. *Journal of Marital and Family Therapy*, 1980, *6*, 55-64.

Gass, G. Z. The role of values in marriage counseling: Comments. *Family Coordinator*, 1970, *19*, 343-345.

Gibbs, H. W., & Achterberg-Lawliss, J. Spiritual values and death anxiety: Implications for counseling with terminal cancer patients. *Journal of Counseling Psychology*, 1978, *25*, 563-569.

Gibran, K. *The prophet.* New York: Knopf, 1923.

Gordon, S. Counselors and changing sexual values. *Personnel and Guidance Journal*, 1976, *54*, 362-364.

Gurman, A. S. The effects and effectiveness of marital therapy: A review of outcome research. *Family Process*, 1973, *12*, 145-170.

Gutsch, K. U. Counseling: The impact of ethics. *Counselor Education and Supervision*, 1968, *7*, 239-243.

Gutsch, K. U., & Rosenblatt, H. S. Counselor education: A touch of Martin Buber's philosophy. *Counselor Education and Supervision*, 1973, *13*, 8-13.

Hammer, M. *The theory and practice of psychotherapy with specific disorders.* Springfield, Ill.: Charles C Thomas, 1972.

Hare-Mustin, R. T. A feminist approach to family therapy. *Family Process*, 1978, *17*, 181-194.

Hinsie, L. E., & Campbell, R. J. *Psychiatric dictionary.* New York: Oxford University Press, 1970.

Hudson, J. W. Value issues in marital counseling. In H. L. Silverman (Ed.), *Marital counseling.* Springfield, Ill.: Charles C Thomas, 1967.

Hulnick, H. R. Counselor: Know thyself. *Counselor Education and Supervision*, 1977, *17*, 69-72.

Hultman, K. E. Values as defenses. *Personnel and Guidance Journal*, 1976, *54*, 268-271.

Kalafat, J., Boroto, D. R., & France, K. Relationships among experience level and value orientation and the performance of paraprofessional telephone counselors. *American Journal of Community Psychology*, 1979, *7*, 167-180.

Kalish, R. A. Of social values and the dying. *Family Coordinator*, 1972, *21*, 81-94.

Kalish, R. A., & Collier, K. W. *Exploring human values: Psychological and philosophical considerations.* Monterey, Calif.: Brooks/Cole, 1981.

Keith, D. V. Use of self: A brief report. *Family Process*, 1974, *13*, 201-206.

Kirkpatrick, J. S. Guidelines for counseling young people with sexual concerns. *Personnel and Guidance Journal*, 1975, *54*, 144-154.

Kremer, E. B., Zimpfer, D. G., & Wiggers, T. T. Homosexuality, counseling, and the adolescent male. *Personnel and Guidance Journal*, 1975, *54*, 94-99.

Lager, E., & Zwerling, I. Time orientation and psychotherapy in the ghetto. *American Journal of Psychiatry*, 1980, *137*, 306-309.

Leslie, G. R. In my own opinion: Personal values, professional ideologies, and family specialists: A new look. *Family Coordinator*, 1979, *28*, 157-162.

Lewis, K. N., & Walsh, W. B. Effects of value-communication style and similarity of values on counselor education. *Journal of Counseling Psychology*, 1980, *27*, 305-314.

Maddock, J. W. Morality and individual development: A basis for value education. *Family Coordinator*, 1972, *21*, 291-302.

Marsh, D. C., & Humphrey, N. D. Value congeries and marriage counseling. *Journal of Marriage and Family Living*, 1953, *15*, 28-34.

Melton, A. W. The marriage counselor and the moral interregnum. *Family Coordinator*, 1968, *17*, 37-40.

Middleton, J. T. The role of values in marriage counseling. *Family Coordinator*, 1970, *19*, 335-341.

Minor, J. H., & Minor, B. J. Value conflict resolution: A training model for counselors of minority clients. *Journal of Employment Counseling*, 1978, *15*, 164-170.

Myers, L. Hyponatology, sex role concepts, and human sexual behavior. *Family Coordinator,* 1973, *22,* 339-344.

Nathanson, R. Counseling persons with disabilities: Are the feelings, thoughts, and behaviors of helping professionals helpful? *Personnel and Guidance Journal,* 1979, *58,* 233-237.

Neubeck, G. Toward a theory of marriage counseling: A humanistic approach. *Family Coordinator,* 1973, *22,* 117-122.

Nichols, W. C. The field of marriage counseling: A brief overview. *Family Coordinator,* 1973, *22,* 3-14.

Nutt, R. L. Review and preview of attitudes and values of counselors of women. *Counseling Psychologist,* 1979, *8,* 18-20.

Peterson, G. B., & Peterson, L. R. Sexism in the treatment of sexual dysfunction. *Family Coordinator,* 1973, *22,* 397-404.

Piel, E. R. A theory of imperfection: An imperfect theory? *Counselor Education and Supervision,* 1979, *19,* 54-59.

Piercy, F., & Schultz, K. Values clarification strategies for couples' enrichment. *Family Coordinator,* 1978, *27,* 175-178.

Polmantier, P. C. Don't compromise on a counselor. *School Executive,* 1947, *67,* 33-34.

Polmantier, P. C. The personality of the counselor. *Vocational Guidance Quarterly,* 1966, *45,* 95-99.

Price-Bonham, S., & Murphy, D. C. Dual-career marriages: Implications for the clinician. *Journal of Marital and Family Therapy,* 1980, *6,* 181-188.

Rice, D. G., Fey, W. F., & Kepecs, J. G. Therapist experience and "style" as factors in co-therapy. *Family Process,* 1972, *11,* 1-12.

Rokeach, M. *The nature of human values.* New York: Free Press, 1973.

Roman, M., Charles, E., & Karasu, T. B. The value systems of psychotherapists and changing mores. *Psychotherapy: Theory, Research, and Practice,* 1978, *15,* 409-445.

Silverman, H. L. Value issues in marriage counseling: Psychological and philosophical implications. *Family Coordinator,* 1973, *22,* 103-110.

Smith, D., & Peterson, J. Counseling and values in a time perspective. *Personnel and Guidance Journal,* 1977, *55,* 309-318. (a)

Smith, D., & Peterson, J. Values: A challenge to the profession. *Personnel and Guidance Journal,* 1977, *55,* 227-231. (b)

Sunbury, J. F. Working with defensive projection in conjoint marriage counseling. *Family Relations,* 1980, *29,* 107-110.

Thompson, G. H., & Fishburn, W. R. Attitudes toward homosexuality among graduate counseling students. *Counselor Education and Supervision,* 1977, *17,* 121-130.

Tsoi-Hoshmand, L. T. Marital therapy and changing values. *Family Coordinator,* 1976, *25,* 51-56.

Walker, B. A., Somerfeld, E., & Robinson, R. One-night stands: A challenge for family therapists. *Family Therapy,* 1978, *5,* 259-265.

Wright, M. R. Psychological aspects of vasectomy counseling. *Family Coordinator,* 1972, *21,* 259-265.

4. Ethical Divorce Therapy and Divorce Proceedings: A Psycholegal Perspective

Florence W. Kaslow, Ph.D.
President
Kaslow Associates, P.A.
Private Practice in Therapy and Consultation
West Palm Beach, Florida

Joseph L. Steinberg, LL.B.
Attorney-at-Law
School of Social Work and School of Law
University of Connecticut
Hartford, Connecticut

Four

ACCOUNTABILITY, PEER REVIEW, STAGES OF NORMAL development à la Kohlberg (1969), and forensic psychology and psychiatry[1] have all catapulted onto center stage in the mental health showcase of the 1970s. Family therapy practice, like all forms of psychotherapeutic practice, has been increasingly regulated by law. To illustrate, most states during the past decade began to require that professionals report cases of suspected child abuse to the designated public authority. The Supreme Court of California, in the much publicized *Tarasoff* case,[2] held that therapists have a "duty to warn" a potential victim of a patient's homicidal intentions, and the dictum was translated in the American Psychological Association's *Monitor* ("California court ruling," 1975) as "privilege ends where peril begins."

A similar duty-to-warn decision was promulgated in a New Jersey case[3] upholding the *Tarasoff* contention that a threat of dangerousness is compelling in its seriousness and that the therapist in effect has a responsibility to apprise the possible victim, thus transcending the professional adherence to the doctrine of confidentiality. Such precedent-setting laws and court decisions have radically altered the practice of psychotherapy, so that many clinicians now debate issues such as (a) What should and should not go into records given the possibility that one might be subpoenaed? (b) Who is the client (Monahan, 1980)? (c) To whom is the therapist responsible—the patient, society, the institution in which he/she functions, the intended victim, or the profession of which he/she is a member? and (d) How much malpractice insurance should be carried?

Even in a totally private, independent practice, the clinician is aware of the dictates of law, the regulation of their profession, and the requirements of third-party insurance payers. Responses to these dilemmas have been codified in professional codes of ethics such as that of the American Psychological Association (APA) (1981) which states the following:

> Principle 7. Professional Relationships
>
> Psychologists act with due regard for the needs, special competencies and obligations of their colleagues in psychology and other professions. They respect the prerogatives and obligations of the institutions or organizations with which these other colleagues are associated.

Another reality factor in the family therapists' professional life is the spiraling number of areas of practice in which it is essential to interface with attorneys and judges. Whether the issue is adoption, custody, child or spouse abuse, involuntary commitment, the privacy rights of a minor in therapy or for abortion on request, testamentary capacity, or euthanasia, to name a few, the therapist is literally thrust into contact with those trained in the law and in the adversary system. Their perspectives are often diametrically opposite. The therapist is educated in the humanistic tradition, attempting to see many facets of the situation and convinced that there is rarely one guilty (or sick) member of the family with all others innocent (or well). Many attorneys conceptualize in terms of guilt and innocence, perpetrator and victim.

Each professional believes he/she is trying to serve the client's best interest, but each may perceive this from a totally different vantage point. For example, the family therapist may believe the explosive, homicidal son in the family he or she is seeing needs to be hospitalized in order to be safely confined while ensuring his "right to treatment" and protecting the rest of the family from his wrath until they can become less provocative. Conversely, the attorney appointed to represent the son at the commitment hearing is more concerned about the young man's desire for and right to liberty. Here the virtues of freedom transcend the powers of medication and institutionalization. The attorney and therapist each are advocates for what they believe is their mutual client's best interest and often find themselves in an adversarial relationship to each other.

It is hoped that the model for respectful interdisciplinary functioning presented here in the context of divorce and child custody cases can be used as a prototype for other situations as well. Lawyers and therapists must cooperate and collaborate on behalf of their mutual clients, and avoid giving them conflicting advice and causing confusion and distress over divided loyalties where areas of professional concern may overlap.

ONE CLIENT UNIT—TWO PROFESSIONALS

There is increasingly a clarion call for cooperation between legal and mental health professionals during a client's divorce (Bernstein, 1976; Kaslow, 1979-1980; Steinberg, 1980). The call has become widespread enough to suggest an emerging new standard for individual practitioners involved in implementing the divorce process. The standard suggests that neither legal nor mental health professionals can consider their efforts complete or their services effective if they have not guided their clients into working relationships with competent practitioners in the other field.[4]

Rephrased, the standard becomes "a legal resolution that ignores the client's psychological needs is as inappropriate as a psychological resolution that conflicts with the client's legal needs. A viable solution can only result from a careful and balanced consideration of the concerns of both disciplines" (Steinberg, 1980, p. 261).

Practitioners who do not assume the responsibility for encouraging and assuring a psycholegal interface for each divorcing client may, by definition, be providing inadequate services. Practitioners whose expertise, however substantial, is limited solely to their own areas of professionalism are likely to be lacking in insights and information necessary for an adequately broad spectrum of professional performance.

Lawyers and therapists whose knowledge of the process of marital dissolution does not include a working familiarity with and appreciation of the other profession's basic precepts may shortchange their clients. The clinician usually focuses on the emotional, affective components of the process; the attorney is and should be primarily concerned with the cognitive aspects—the legal and economic ramifications (Bohannan, 1973). Often, neither has a full sense of the interplay between these dimensions. For example, the couple may quarrel incessantly about who is to get a painting, holding up the proceedings for months while they haggle. Financially, it may not be very valuable, and so the argument does not make much sense economically. But emotionally the painting may have been selected with loving care by the couple and may represent a treasured memory with which neither cares to part. They may also need this additional time of arguing as a prelude to the final parting. Only when attorney and therapist can be in contact and have a modicum of trust in each other's good intentions, competence, and interpretive astuteness can they comprehend the hologram (Duhl, 1981) and fathom the larger scene that evolves from fitting the puzzle pieces together.

There is a possibility that to not collaborate might constitute malpractice. The American Bar Association Code of Professional Responsibility, Ethical Consideration 7-8 (1970), states the following:

> A lawyer should exert his (her) best efforts to insure that decisions of his (her) client are made only after the client has been informed of relevant considerations. A lawyer ought to initiate this decision-making process if the client does not do so. Advice of a lawyer to his (her) client need not be confined to purely legal consideration.

Certainly, this ethical consideration offers a substantial basis for suggesting that legal issues surrounding custody require clients to be informed by their attorney about relevant studies of the impact of divorce on children of dissolving families. Hetherington (1972); Gardner (1976); Hetherington, Cox, and Cox (1977); McDermott (1968); and Wallerstein and Kelly (1979, 1980) are a few of the mental health professionals whose publications should become familiar to matrimonial lawyers and their clients. Their research reports the ill effects of the trauma of divorce and the generally negative impact of parental loss on children of all ages.

The Ethical Considerations found in the American Bar Association's Code of Professional Responsibility seem to move even further by suggesting, in part, in that same paragraph, Ethical Consideration 7-8:

> In assisting his (her) client to reach a proper decision, it is often desirable for a lawyer to point out those factors which may lead to a decision which is morally just as well as legally permissible. He (she) may emphasize the possibility of harsh consequences that might result from assertion of legally permissible positions.

Certainly, psychologically inadvisable attempts to severely restrict visitation privileges may do serious damage to the noncustodial parent as well as to the children. The California Child Custody Act of 1979 espouses the principle that whenever possible children should have equal access to both parents. Spouses may sever their marital bonds, but divorce does not terminate the role of either or their function as a parent. Children need to know that both parents are still concerned about and involved in their life and should be spared as much as possible the bitterness and recriminations in which their parents may engage. They should be helped to realize that they did not cause the breakup, nor could they have prevented it from occurring. The decision was made by the adults.

A vengeful economic war may have consequences beyond the courtroom that can color the dissolving family's future. Take, for example, the situation in which the husband's extramarital affairs have become obvious to the wife. His ongoing philandering becomes intolerable. They have entered conjoint divorce therapy. In the first six sessions, as the marital relationship appears irreparable, the focus has been on disentangling their neurotic interaction as they work toward physical separation and ultimately a constructive divorce. He has rented an apartment and is ready to move. Then he consults an attorney who, perhaps, tells him, "Do not move yet; it is cheaper to stay there and only pay one rent and no support payments. By keeping the pressure on her, she'll buckle more quickly and agree to a settlement and payments that will be much lower." This convincing economic argument often prevails over the therapeutic logic about psychological well-being, and he continues to live in the household where the tension escalates, the children get more entangled in the fray, and their anger at one or both parents for the torture accumulates.

By the time the matter gets to court, after numerous delays occasioned by burgeoning court calendars or tactical advantage seeking, a private decision to separate has become a major public battle in which the two members of the family most affected often abdicate their psychological wishes and needs in favor of an adversarial process and maneuvers. The psychic scars for ex-spouses and their offspring take long to heal; the pain continues well after the actual legal contest ends and the attorney is long since out of the picture. This impinges on formal custody and visitation arrangements and may cause deep seated hostile feelings in children towards parents.

Obviously, an inequitable settlement keeps the parties embattled and embittered and does not permit them to bring the psychic divorce to closure and to re-equilibrate (Kaslow, 1981). The children often become trophies with economic value ascribed to them in the continuing divorce war. Attorneys and therapists both should seek to prevent such a travesty.

The American Bar Association's Ethical Consideration 7-8 suggests that (*infra*) matrimonial lawyers may well have a professional responsibility to become familiar with the tragic consequences of continued battling reported in the psychological literature and by casualties of such warfare and to emphasize these while offering sound legal counsel that considers the whole person—not just the economic aspects.

An emerging legal requirement, suggesting an obligation to provide competent psychological counseling during marital dissolution, is found in another Ethical Consideration of the Code, 6-3, which reads in part that a

> lawyer generally should not accept employment in any area of the law in which he (she) is not qualified. However, he (she) may accept such employment if, in good faith, he (she) expects to become qualified through study and investigations. . . . Proper preparation and representation may require the association by the lawyer of professionals in other disciplines.

Obviously, the professionals of other disciplines will often be mental health and family therapy practitioners—particularly when the issues are rooted in family dilemmas.

The same professional caveats apply to therapists involved with clients going through a divorce. The pragmatic issue, of course, is how therapists can best achieve the attitudes, insights, and information that lead to the necessary interdisciplinary collaborative skills. In addition to reading books and journals, attendance at forensic workshops and lectures and seeking consultative arrangements with attorneys are possibilities. Certainly at a minimum a clinician should obtain and become conversant with appropriate state legislation and major court decisions on divorce and custody. These constitute prime illustrations of situations in which ignorance of the law is no excuse. To practice in the delicate area of divorce and postdivorce therapy without familiarity with the legal regulations violates professional standards of practice and may also be construed as malpractice. For example, the American Psychological Association (APA),[5] in its 1979 version of Ethical Standards for Psychologists, states in Principle 2 (Competence) that

> the maintenance of high standards of professional competence is a responsibility shared by all psychologists in the interest of

the public and the profession as a whole. Psychologists recognize the boundaries of their competence and the limitations of their techniques and only provide services, use techniques, or offer opinions as professionals that meet recognized standards. Psychologists maintain knowledge of current scientific and professional information related to the services they render.

It becomes clear that family and divorce therapists should acquire, at the least, a rudimentary knowledge of the legal areas involved in divorce such as custody, taxation, insurance, and real estate. They should also develop an understanding of the basic thrusts of the statutes that control the legal process of divorce. An awareness of the underlying philosophical principles that govern the courts in settling disputes is also essential. For example, they must understand such concepts as the best interests of the child, equitable distribution of property, and marital fault. It is imperative to know the major provisions of the state's divorce code.

In an earlier example, we wrote of the attorney who advises a husband not to move out because it is much less costly to stay at home. Today the opposite advice is often given because in some states where no-fault divorce laws prevail, time needed to be eligible for divorce is computed from the day the couple physically separated to live in different places. Any further cohabitation nullifies time already accumulated. If the attorney recommends a rapid moving out because of such legal stipulations while the therapist is encouraging them to stay together a little longer as they still seem to care and in part would like to resolve their disagreements, then they are working at cross-purposes and confusing the client. If the therapist lacks pertinent knowledge of the state's divorce code, he or she is functioning in a legal vacuum and is making an egregious error in practice.

Clinicians should also be well informed regarding such concepts as confidentiality, privilege, and informed consent. These are particularly thorny issues if the therapist has originally seen a couple for marital therapy. Later, when they decide to divorce, one of the parties may waive privilege and ask his or her attorney to contact the therapist for his or her records or to testify in a custody hearing. The other partner may refuse—holding the therapist to the guarantee of confidentiality. Critical concerns such as who is considered to be the patient, what records to bring when one receives a subpoena duces tecum, and how much the therapist should and must disclose (Lifshutz, 1970) under any given set of circumstances must be attended to. The therapist, who may be treating both spouses and knows that conjoint or concurrent treatment is ethical and often advisable, may find that a lawyer is forbidden to represent both clients and that each spouse must hire separate legal counsel. Such facts must be checked and accepted, even if the therapist personally disagrees with an adversarial model.

While pursuing these concerns and points of information, it is not essential that the therapist attempt to achieve mastery of these areas. He or she remains a clinician and does not need to become equipped to practice law. To become and remain informed poses a real challenge, since the law is constantly changing legislatively, judicially, and communally. In-depth knowledge and comprehension require law school training and a continuous detailed immersion in statutory changes and in the weekly flow of judicial decisions. To remain abreast also requires regular courtroom appearances to ensure an appreciation of the subtle alterations that occur on an almost daily basis, plus frequent interactions with other attorneys to be familiar with current values and attitudes in the field. This is the prerogative and bailiwick of the attorney, not of the clinician.

Certainly though, therapists can and should avail themselves of workshops and conferences sponsored by local, state, and national bar organizations, papers published in law journals, and texts published within the field. Similarly, attorneys should peruse the books and journals focusing on family dynamics and functioning, divorce and custody, and attend relevant workshops under the aegis of mental health professionals. But, they should not seek to be the therapist—this takes graduate education and advanced clinical training.

By entering into dialogue with professionals in the other field, each can be apprised of what educational opportunities exist. Attending a program in the other discipline will begin a process that will result in one's name appearing on multiple mailing lists. Within months, through the magic of computerized addressing equipment and the incestuous nature of continuing educational programs, one is likely to become the harried recipient of multiple and enticing invitations.

Next, it is possible to develop a local interdisciplinary network. In Philadelphia, for example, the first author belonged to the Community Service Institute, a group comprised of attorneys, judges, and therapists of various disciplines. This organization convenes monthly for dinner followed by a preplanned lecture or panel on topics of vital mutual interest. The dynamic flow of information and the informal opportunity to exchange ideas and become acquainted outside of litigious circumstances open the avenues for the more enlightened understanding and potential collaborations being advocated here. From such interactions, both attorneys and therapists can build referral lists of individuals in the companion discipline to whom they can comfortably and ethically refer clients.

Another source of information about potential referrals is the satisfied client. Having acquired names of likely referral sources in this way, one can call and invite the professional to lunch, sharing the laudatory comments of the client as the basis for the call. Although the recipient of the call may react with surprise, the luncheon invitation is often accepted.

Within months of beginning such an "awareness campaign," one may have spoken to and perhaps lunched with half a dozen sterling practitioners and may have developed a mutually beneficial network.

Having done some or all of the above, a therapist becomes able to actively participate in his or her client's choice of an appropriate divorce lawyer. Few experiences are quite as sad or disheartening as working assiduously with troubled clients heading toward divorce only to have all of one's efforts to help the client achieve emotional stability and utilize the divorce process as a constructive experience undermined by (the choice of) an inappropriate adversarial attorney.

To ignore the client's need for competent legal counsel and leave the distressed client's choice to chance may well be unprofessional. (A similar process of acquiring a list of excellent therapists who specialize in family and divorce therapy would be equally valuable to the attorney, of course.)

CONCLUSION

Individuals whose general pattern of coping with adversity is to become emotionally disabled are often unable to progress through the stages of the divorce process (Bohannan, 1973; Kaslow, 1981; Kessler, 1975). These individuals rarely recover from the debilitating effects of divorce.

> Their lives remain filled with loneliness, self-pity, and unresolved anger as they cling to the inglorious past, unwilling to fashion a meaningful present. Periodically relitigating custody or support orders, these persons use such litigation as occasions to convince friends and family to side with them and to reassure

themselves of the validity of their position. Sadly, they also often attempt to convince their children that the ex-spouse wronged them and they expect their children to behave in ways which will compensate them for their self-inflicted suffering (Kaslow, 1979–1980, p. 75).

A sensitive, humane attorney can try to defuse the continued efforts at retaliation and help the client leave the past and live in the present.

The basic roles of the attorney and therapist are sharply defined. The attorney seeks to protect the client's legal and economic interests while the therapist attempts to help the patient regain functional autonomy. Nonetheless, there may be much overlap in their provision of services. We have attempted to provide attorney and therapist alike with a shared awareness of the psycholegal effects of the divorce process that will allow them to better serve the clients. Such information should enable professionals from both disciplines to generalize to the divorcing person about the emotional as well as legal consequences of the divorce experience. These data will serve to reassure a client about the normalcy of his or her uncertainties, fears, and other psychological reactions. Such knowledge will also allow all involved to better explain the potential reverberations of different plans of action so that the client will be able to make judicious decisions.

Divorce is a traumatic and baffling experience. It marks the destruction of dreams of marital happiness and permanence and unfortunately is often interpreted to represent personal failure, lack of commitment, and poor judgment.

The attorney and the therapist are society's two representatives designated to assist the divorcing through this turbulent time. To ensure that they receive the highest quality professional services, it is essential that the members of both disciplines be acquainted with each other's area of expertise and be willing to consult and cooperate on behalf of the client (Kaslow, 1979–1980, p. 17).

They may even find the interaction personally stimulating and fruitful, as we have. As indicated earlier, failure to do so may be construed as a form of malpractice.

NOTES

[1] Both forensic psychology and forensic psychiatry established boards in 1977 to examine the expertise of their practitioners and to board certify as diplomates the most outstanding members of these specialties.

[2] Tarasoff v. Regents of the University of California, 17 Cal.3d, 425, 131 Cal. Rptr. 14, 551 P.2d334 (1976).

[3] McIntosh v. Milano, 168 N.J. Super. 466, 403A.2d, 500 (N.J. Super., Law Div., 1979).

[4] The negotiation or arbitration of divorce disputes has also moved into prominence in the past decade. These approaches, as well as Coogler's (1978) structured mediation model, offer viable alternatives, in some cases, to the traditional legal adversarial model.

[5] APA is used generically. The other mental health professions hold to similar canons of ethics.

REFERENCES

American Bar Association. *Code of professional responsibility, ethical consideration* 7-8, 1970.

American Psychological Association. *Ethical principles of psychologists* (Rev. ed.). Washington, D.C.: Author, 1981.

Bernstein, B. Lawyer and counselor as an interdisciplinary team: The timely referral. *Journal of Marriage and Family Counseling,* 1976, *2,* 247–354.

Bohannan, P. The six stations of divorce. In M.E. Lasswell & T.E. Lasswell (Eds.), *Love, marriage and family: A developmental approach.* Glenview, Ill.: Scott, Foresman, 1973.

California court ruling on dangerousness stirs controversy. *APA Monitor,* March 1975, pp. 5–6.

Coogler, O.J. *Structured mediation in divorce settlement.* Lexington, Mass.: Lexington Books, 1978.

Duhl, F. The use of the chronological chart in general systems family therapy. *Journal of Marital and Family Therapy,* 1981, *7,* 361–374.

Gardner, R.A. *Psychotherapy with children of divorce.* New York: Aronson, 1976.

Hetherington, E.M. Effects of fathers' absence on personality development in adolescent daughters. *Developmental Psychology,* 1972, *7,* 313–326.

Hetherington, E.M., Cox, M., & Cox, R. The aftermath of divorce. In J.H. Stevens, Jr. & M. Matthews (Eds.), *Mother-child, father-child relations.* Washington, D.C.: National Association for the Education of Young Children, 1977.

In re Lifshutz, Cal. 3d 415, 467 P.2d 557, 85 California Reporter, 829 (1970).

Kaslow, F.W. Stages of divorce: A pscholegal perspective. *Villanova Law Review,* 1979–1980, *25,* 718–751.

Kaslow, F.W. Divorce and divorce therapy. In A. Gurman & D. Kniskern (Eds.), *Handbook of family therapy.* New York: Brunner/Mazel, 1981.

Kessler, S. *The American way of divorce: Prescription for change.* Chicago: Nelson-Hall, 1975.

Kohlberg, L. Stage and sequence: The cognitive developmental approach to socialization. In D.A. Goslin (Ed.), *Handbook of socialization theory and research.* New York: Rand McNally, 1969.

McDermott, J.F. Parental divorce in early childhood. *American Journal of Psychiatry,* 1968, *124,* 1424–1432.

Monahan, J. *Who is the client?* Washington, D.C.: American Psychological Association, 1980.

Steinberg, J.L. Towards an interdisciplinary commitment: A divorce lawyer proposes attorney-therapist marriages or, at the least, an affair. *Journal of Marital and Family Therapy,* 1980, *6,* 259–268.

Wallerstein, J.S., & Kelly, J.B. Divorce and children. In J.D. Noshpitz (Ed.), *Handbook of child psychiatry IV.* New York: Basic Books, 1979.

Wallerstein, J.S., & Kelly, J.B. *Surviving the breakup: How children and parents cope with divorce.* New York: Basic Books, 1980.

5. Ethical Conflict in Clinical Decision Making: A Challenge for Family Therapists

James K. Morrison, Ph.D.
Clinical Psychologist
Department of Psychiatry
Albany Medical College
Albany, New York

Bruce Layton, Ph.D.
Institute for Program Evaluation
U. S. General Accounting Office
Washington, D.C.

Joan Newman, Ph.D.
Child Research and Study Center
State University of New York at Albany
Albany, New York

Five

ACCORDING TO HOBBS (1965) ETHICS IS NOT JUST A GUIDE to conduct but "the very essence of the treatment process itself" (p. 1508). In the same vein, London (1977) asserts that one can no longer question the powerful influence of the therapists' values but can only determine the way in which those values are permitted to influence the therapeutic transaction. If ethical concerns are at the heart of the psychotherapeutic process, it seems unfortunate that family therapists have devoted so little attention to such concerns in the literature. This lack of emphasis on ethical issues involved in therapy is also reflected in the lack of systematic ethics training in most graduate programs as well as in the growing involvement of the courts in resolving conflicts between clients and therapists (Hines & Hare-Mustin, 1978).

Mailloux (1977) emphasizes the need among all psychotherapists to adopt a value-oriented approach to the delivery of services to clients. According to Mailloux, simply conceptualizing family therapy as a problem-solving intervention is too narrow an approach. The ethical issues surrounding such interventions as family therapy can no longer be ignored because the professional and personal values that give direction to family therapists' interventions may conflict not just with one person's value system but with those of the entire family.

ETHICAL ISSUES WITHIN THE GENERAL CLINICAL FIELD

In the past decade we have witnessed a proliferation of ethical issues emerging from the whole mental health arena. Due to the lack of attention to such issues among family therapists, it would be well to review the literature in the general mental health field where ethical issues have aroused considerable interest. Open debate over these ethical issues seems to have increased the conflict experienced by clinicians to the extent that certain clinical decisions (e.g., recommending involuntary hospitalization) can generate a great deal of anxiety. Clinicians actively engaged in the delivery of mental health services must at some point come to terms with ethical issues to best protect the rights of clients, as well as to achieve a resolution of personal conflict over such issues. A closer look at issues not often raised in family therapy literature would seem pertinent.

A variety of ethical issues have been delineated in the literature. Mental health professionals have been accused of becoming unwitting agents of the establishment (Beit-Hallahmi, 1974; Halleck, 1971; Mancuso, Eson, & Morrison, 1979; Redlich & Mollica, 1976; Szasz, 1970a, 1970b), and of not taking adequate steps to preserve the confidentiality of information revealed by clients (Brodsky, 1972; Morrison, Federico, & Rosenthal, 1975; Redlich & Mollica, 1976). Furthermore, such clinicians have been excoriated for excluding mental patients and inmates from access to clinical records (Brodsky, 1972).

Perhaps the most heated controversy derives from charges by some that certain clinical interventions are immoral. Psychosurgery, electroshock treatment, involuntary commitment to a mental hospital, and the forced injection of unwilling patients with psychopharmacologic agents have been severely critized by some individuals on grounds that such interventions are not only immoral but of questionable efficacy and legality as well (M. Glenn, 1974; Older, 1974; Redlich & Mollica, 1976; Szasz, 1970a).

The process of making psychiatric diagnoses also has been severely questioned due to the unreliability and stigma often associated with the process (Rosenhan, 1973, 1975). Finally, some (e.g., Morrison & Gaviria, 1979) question the ethics of promoting the use of mental health procedures in other spheres of influence (e.g., politics, law, etc.).

Ethical Concerns about Children and Adolescents

There has recently been a rapidly increasing interest among mental health professionals in the ethical issues raised by the delivery of therapeutic services to children. Ethical issues raised by such professionals include the following questions: Is it ethical for parents or legal guardians to be able to coerce their children into psychiatric treatment or hospitalization without their voluntary and informed consent (Beyer & Wilson, 1976)? Is it ethical for a therapist to inform legally responsible parties of information obtained from the child during treatment, even though such information would be deemed privileged and confidential if obtained from an adult (McGuire, 1974)? Issues such as these are often extremely important, given the evidence that children may be medicated for disorders (e.g., minimal brain dysfunction) that are of questionable validity (Moore & Glickstein, 1970; Pond, 1967; Schrag & Divoky, 1976), given psychosurgery unnecessarily (Older, 1974), institutionalized without sufficient cause (Beyer & Wilson, 1976), and, of course, pressured to engage in family therapy when it is obvious that the person does *not* want to cooperate.

Some (Holdridge-Crane, Morrison, & Morrison, 1979) contend that there are solutions to be found to such problems by changing or reinterpreting the laws on informed consent, use of child advocates, more explanations to the family of the need for a service (e.g., family therapy) offered to a child (Koocher, 1976), and more sharing of ethical problems concerning children among mental health professionals.

In recent years there has been a steady shift in therapeutic focus away from seeing the child as the identified client to viewing the child's symptoms as a sign of family pathology. This approach might suggest that the identified client might be the family, not the child. Goggin and Goggin (1979) suggest that using family therapy instead of other forms of therapy seems justified when the child's problem is a manifestation of family interaction. Another indication for family therapy is when the referred child has been scapegoated. However, family therapists in such situations must face the often difficult task of conveying to parents that the family has the problem, not the child. This whole issue raises the thorny ethical problem of "blaming." A family therapist must try to avoid blaming either the child or the whole family. Furthermore, as Hines and Hare-Mustin (1978) and Minuchin (1974) point out, requiring all family members to participate in family therapy may not always be in an identified client's best interests.

Ethics and Behavior Therapy

Some behaviorally oriented psychotherapists have been accused of trying to ignore the ethical issues raised by their behavioral interventions

(Kitchener, 1980a). In recent years behavior therapists have devoted more and more attention to discussing the ethical issues surrounding behavior modification (see summary by Begelman, 1975). Recently, some (Houts & Krasner, 1980; Ward, 1980) have tried to counter the arguments of Kitchener (1980b, 1980c). Such debates on ethical issues should be applauded, and it is hoped that the family therapists as a group might engage in the same type of debate.

ETHICAL ISSUES AND FAMILY THERAPY

A number of specific ethical concerns thrust themselves into the work of family therapists. First, whose interest is the therapist ethically bound to serve? Should the therapist who begins working with one client try to involve that person's whole family? What is done in the case of the reluctant adolescent or child? The issue of informed consent is thus raised as an issue that requires, because of its moral and legal ramifications, careful consideration by the family therapist.

Second, should the family therapist attempt to have families reveal all their secrets (e.g., infidelities, criminal records, etc.), even to the extent that some family members may suffer embarrassment, great anxiety, and a loss of respect in the eyes of other members of the family? Mariner (1971) believes that all family members should agree prior to therapy whether information revealed by one family member to the therapist should subsequently be made known to the rest of the family. However, certain types of information may be excluded from that contract. For example, families should realize that therapists may be held legally liable if they do not disclose any client's intent to kill someone else.

Third, therapists working with families should be careful in labeling families as resistant or poor risks for therapy. Thus, before labeling, such therapists should carefully consider how their expectations and biases may prevent them from working with families with whom other therapists with different orientations might well be successful. Family therapists should examine the long-term significance of the labels they use and the extent to which these labels follow from an inability of certain therapists to deal effectively with value systems different from their own.

Another ethical issue of concern to family therapists is raised by Zuk (1972), who points out the possible abuse by a side-taking therapist who uses a position of power to foment conflict or to undercut some family members in the interests of some further solution purportedly for the entire family. Sometimes, family therapists overlook the fact that different members benefit unequally from family therapy.

Hare-Mustin (1980) warns that "family therapy may be dangerous for your health" (p. 395) because family therapists do not always warn their clients of the risks involved in doing family therapy. The priority given to the good of the family as a whole can lead to risks for individuals. By being persuaded to participate in family therapy, individuals may have to subordinate their own goals and give up limited privacy and confidentiality. Even the acceptance of the traditional family as the ideal family model for therapy can foster stereotyped roles that are a disadvantage to certain individuals.

Hines and Hare-Mustin (1978) make recommendations in addressing the type of ethical concerns just mentioned. First, ethical training ought to become an integral part of professional training programs for family therapists. Second, seminars, workshops, and in-service training programs should be used by centers, institutions, and other service agencies to facilitate discussion and development of feasible ethical guidelines.

Family therapists are thus presently faced with an enormous challenge (i.e., coping with a cornucopia of thorny ethical issues that impinge on their work). Because of the more complex nature of their work, family therapists may face more ethical conflicts in their clinical decision making than most other therapists. For example, a family therapist is constantly faced with the question as to whose agent he or she is? Some individual therapists may struggle with the dilemma of whether they are agents of the client or the state (e.g., as in the case of hospital commitment), but family therapists are further faced with accusations that they may be agents of the parents against the children, the children against the parents, or of one parent against the other.

A SURVEY OF ETHICAL CONFLICTS AMONG CLINICIANS

Despite the importance of ethical issues and the conflict they sometimes induce, no investigation of the degree of ethical conflict that various clinical personnel experience has been forthcoming. It is with cognizance of the importance of ethical issues in general clinical work that the authors began a survey of ethical issues and the conflict emerging from them. Although the study focuses on general clinical issues, a brief discussion of the results yields some implications for family therapists as well.

The study focused not just on ethical issues, but on the ethical conflict experienced by the worker. Whether more or less ethical conflict is desirable is, of course, open to question. Some argue that, in spite of the discomfort, mental health workers should make themselves aware of the moral and ethical traps that they have laid for themselves (Mancuso et al., 1979; Morrison & Gaviria, 1979; Szasz, 1970a). Certainly, family therapists and clinicians who place a great deal of emphasis on the value of personal autonomy and dignity would argue that interventions that involve more radical treatment should be undertaken only after the therapist has agonized over the necessity of the intervention.

Thirty-eight clinical psychologists, 41 psychiatrists, 29 psychiatric social workers, 23 psychiatric nurses, and 33 other mental health workers (vocational rehabilitation counselors and mental health therapy aides were combined due to the small numbers in each group) comprised the sample. The 88 males and 76 females had a mean age of 35.4 years and a median of 4.9 years of clinical experience.

The mental health workers from a tri-city area of upstate New York completed the Ethical Conflict Questionnaire (ECQ), a 20-item, reliable ($r = .84$), self-report attitude measure, by providing some biographical information and by responding anonymously to 20 statements reflecting current ethical issues in mental health. Respondents were asked to indicate the degree of ethical conflict that they felt about each issue on a 7-point scale. The degree of experienced conflict ranged from "no conflict," with a scale value of 1, to "extreme conflict," with a scale value of 7. An example of one of the items is the following: "The possibility that you may be imposing middle class values on some of your patients."

Findings

Experience

The results indicated that those mental health workers with more clinical experience reported less overall ethical conflict than those with less clinical experience. Increased clinical experience may thus either bring more expertise to the resolving of ethical conflicts or more skill at actively ignoring the moral aspects of clinical work. At this point, one cannot ascertain which possibilities have the most explanatory value.

Occupations

Generally, among all respondents, clinical psychologists reported the most conflict over ethical issues. Specific attention was given to the contrast between the ethical conflict experienced by psychologists and psychiatrists. A data analysis indicated that clinical psychologists reported significantly more conflict than psychiatrists regarding those procedures that are usually performed by physicians (i.e., making diagnoses, giving tranquilizers, and involuntary hospital commitments of the nondangerous). It would almost appear as if psychologists reported conflict over those clinical interventions for which they seldom have the primary responsibility. By way of contrast, it would appear that since they are asked to undertake many of these clinical interventions, psychiatrists have learned to resolve, in some fashion, conflict over the ethical issues impacting on these interventions.

There was a significant difference in the conflict experienced by psychiatrists and psychologists from that experienced by social workers and nurses. Social workers and nurses reported less conflict involving "involuntary commitment" and "expanding their sphere of influence" but higher conflict involving formal diagnoses.

The rehabilitation counselors and mental health therapy aides differed from psychiatrists, psychologists, nurses, and social workers in that they reported significantly less conflict regarding interventions in which they were seldom directly involved (e.g., making a formal diagnosis and encouraging the use of tranquilizers). Such responses probably reflect the decreased responsibility that such professionals feel, at least by comparison, with those mental health workers more directly involved in such interventions.

Sex

Sex of the mental health worker also influenced the degree of reported ethical conflict. However, occupation as a psychiatrist or a psychologist made a larger difference in the amount of experienced conflict among females than among males. As a result, female psychiatrists apparently experience a great deal more ethical conflict than do female psychologists, whereas, among males, psychiatrists report slightly less conflict than do psychologists. The results may be attributable to the different ways in which professional conflicts are resolved by men and women, or the actual work roles and associated ethical dilemmas of men and women may be different, even within the same professional occupation group.

Although the findings cannot be explained, it is obvious that there is an interaction effect between sex and occupation.

The ECQ did not elicit unidimensional responses related to ethical conflict. For example, the mental health workers reported high conflict on some issues and low conflict on others. This implies that although some individuals may experience consistently high or low conflict, most therapists feel differently about different ethical issues.

Implications

A number of considerations emerge from this study. First, it is important for the therapist to be aware of his/her attitudes regarding various ethical issues. Although the survey shows some variations among occupations, sex, and experience, it comes down to the individual therapist with the client family and a specific issue. Increased emphasis on ethical issues can be included in family therapy training. It is also important for therapists in clinical settings to discuss ethical issues. Although this survey found differences in ethical concerns among different occupational groups, it would be difficult to assign families or even permit them a choice of professional.

The sex of the therapist could be discussed with the family. Since sex may be an important factor in certain ethical issues, the family may want to have cotherapists, one of each sex. In clinics where it is feasible, families may have the option of selecting a more experienced therapist. However, this survey did not show that experienced therapists would make better resolutions, only that they had less decision-making conflict.

From the presenting problem and intake information, family therapists may begin to discuss prior to therapy the ethical issues that may affect a family during the course of family therapy. Such discussions could foster the matching of therapist(s) to families with the minimum amount of risk of ethical conflict. Family therapy is difficult enough without ethical conflicts providing unnecessary interference.

Clearly, this survey of ethical conflicts needs to be repeated with a population of family therapists to determine whether sex, years of clinical experience, and occupation affect the degree of ethical conflict. Furthermore, there is a need to develop another version of the ECQ that would address ethical issues of special relevance to family therapists. Such a version, administered to both family and therapists, would facilitate interesting research and may be used by the family and therapist in the therapeutic process.

Finally, because of the importance of ethical conflicts in the treatment of families, family therapists might consider the value of a consumer approach to families (Hare-Mustin, Marecek, Kaplan, & Liss-Levinson, 1979; Morrison, 1978; 1979a; 1979b). Such an approach, already successful in community psychology and among individual psychotherapy clients in private practice, might enable family therapists to better implement some of the recommendations made in this article.

REFERENCES

Begelman, D.A. Ethical and legal issues of behavior modification. In M. Hersen, R.M. Eisler, & P.M. Miller (Eds.), *Progress in behavior modification* (Vol. 1). New York: Academic Press, 1975.

Beit-Hallahmi, B. Salvation and its vicissitudes: Clinical psychology and political values. *American Psychologist,* 1974, *29,* 124–129.

Beyer, H.A., & Wilson, J.P. The reluctant volunteer: A child's right to resist commitment. In E.P. Koocher (Ed.), *Children's rights and the mental health professions.* New York: Wiley, 1976.

Brodsky, S.L. Shared results and open files with the client. *Professional Psychology,* 1972, *4,* 362–364.

Glenn, M. *Voices from the asylum.* New York: Harper & Row, 1974.

Goggin, J., & Goggin, E. When adult therapists work with children: Differential treatment considerations. *Professional Psychology,* 1979, *10,* 330–332.

Halleck, S.L. *The politics of therapy.* New York: Science House, 1971.

Hare-Mustin, R.T. Family therapy may be dangerous for your health. *Professional Psychology,* 1980, *11,* 935–938.

Hare-Mustin, R.T., Maracek, J., Kaplan, A.G., & Liss-Levinson, N. Rights of clients, responsibilities of therapists. *American Psychologist,* 1979, *34,* 3–16.

Hines, P.M., & Hare-Mustin, R.T. Ethical concerns in family therapy. *Professional Psychology,* 1978, *9,* 165–171.

Hobbs, N. Ethics in clinical psychology. In B. Wolman (Ed.), *Handbook in clinical psychology.* New York: McGraw-Hill, 1965.

Holdridge-Crane, S., Morrison, K.L., & Morrison, J.K. The child-consumer's informed consent to treatment: Ethical, psychological and legal implications. In J.K. Morrison (Ed.), *A consumer approach to community psychology.* Chicago: Nelson-Hall, 1979.

Houts, A.C., & Krasner, L. Slicing the ethical Gordian knot: A response to Kitchener. *Journal of Consulting and Clinical Psychology,* 1980, *48,* 8–10.

Kitchener, R.F. Ethical relativism and behavior therapy. *Journal of Consulting and Clinical Psychology,* 1980, *48,* 1–7. (a)

Kitchener, R.F. Ethical relativism, ethical naturalism, and behavior therapy. *Journal of Consulting and Clinical Psychology,* 1980, *48,* 14–16. (b)

Kitchener, R.F. Ethical skepticism and behavior therapy: A reply to Ward. *Journal of Consulting and Clinical Psychology,* 1980, *48,* 649–651. (c)

Koocher, R. (Ed.), *Children's rights and the mental health professions.* New York: Wiley, 1976.

London, P. *Behavior control* (2nd ed.). New York: New American Library, 1977.

Mancuso, J.C., Eson, M.E., & Morrison, J.K. Psychology in the morals market place: Role dilemma for community psychologists. In J.K. Morrison (Ed.), *A consumer approach to community psychology.* Chicago: Nelson-Hall, 1979.

McGuire, J.M. Confidentiality and the child in psychotherapy. *Professional Psychology,* 1974, *5,* 372-379.

Mailloux, N. Ethical issues in the psychologist-client relationship. *International Journal of Psychology,* 1977, *16,* 115-119.

Mariner, A. Psychotherapists' communication with patient's relatives and referring professionals. *American Journal of Psychotherapy,* 1971, *25,* 517-529.

Minuchin, S. *Families and family therapy.* Cambridge, Mass.: Harvard University Press, 1974.

Moore, R.Y., & Glickstein, M. Biological factors in development. In H.W. Reese & L.P. Lipsitt (Eds.), *Experimental child psychology.* New York: Academic Press, 1970.

Morrison, J.K. The client as consumer and evaluation of community mental health services. *American Journal of Community Psychology,* 1978, *6,* 147-155.

Morrison, J.K. *A consumer approach to community psychology.* Chicago: Nelson-Hall, 1979. (a)

Morrison, J.K. A consumer-oriented approach to psychotherapy. *Psychotherapy: Theory, Research and Practice,* 1979, *16,* 381-384. (b)

Morrison, J.K., Federico, M., & Rosenthal, H.J. Contracting confidentiality in group psychotherapy. *Journal of Forensic Psychology,* 1975, *7,* 1-6.

Morrison, J.K., & Gaviria, B. The role of the client-consumer in the delivery of psychiatric services. In J.K. Morrison (Ed.), *A consumer approach to community psychology.* Chicago: Nelson-Hall, 1979.

Older, J. Psychosurgery: Ethical issues and a proposal for control. *American Journal of Orthopsychiatry,* 1974, *44,* 661-674.

Pond, D. Behavior disorders in brain-damaged children. In D. Williams (Ed.), *Modern trends in neurology.* (Series 4), Washington, D.C.: Butterworth, 1967.

Redlich, F., & Mollica, R.F. Overview: Ethical issues in contemporary psychiatry. *American Journal of Psychiatry,* 1976, *133,* 125-136.

Rosenhan, D.L. On being sane in insane places. *Science,* 1973, *179,* 250-258.

Rosenhan, D.L. The contextual nature of psychiatric diagnoses. *Journal of Abnormal Psychology,* 1975, *84,* 462-474.

Schrag, P., & Divoky, D. *The myth of the hyperactive child and other means of child control.* New York: Pantheon Books, 1976.

Szasz, T.S. *Ideology and insanity.* New York: Doubleday, 1970. (a)

Szasz, T.S. *The manufacture of madness.* New York: Delta, 1970. (b)

Ward, L.C. Behavior therapy and ethics: A response to Kitchener. *Journal of Consulting and Clinical Psychology,* 1980, *48,* 646-648.

Zuk, G.R. Family therapy: Clinical hodgepodge or clinical science. *Journal of Marriage and Family Counseling,* 1972, *2,* 229-304.

6. Ignorance of the Law Is No Excuse

Barton E. Bernstein, M.L.A., J.D.
Attorney-at-Law
Adjunct Assistant Professor of Psychiatry
Southwestern Medical School
Dallas, Texas

Adjunct Associate Professor
University of Texas
Graduate School of Social Work
Arlington, Texas

Six

"IGNORANTIA LEGIS EXCUSAT NEMINEM." THIS PHRASE, attributed to John Selden (1584-1654), is prominently emblazoned in marble, wood, or plastic in every law school in the country. Law students are reminded to heed the warning during exam time, and even the general public is reminded of its import during civil and criminal trials of every nature, when their rights and the rights of others or the state are involved. Yet therapists, dealing with people and feelings, often are intimidated by the law, lawyers, and the effect of either or both on their clients and themselves.

Although a few therapeutic training curriculums (psychiatry, psychology, social work, marriage and family counseling, pastoral counseling, psychotherapy, etc.) have a solid base of substantive and procedural legal knowledge, there is a paucity of technical legal knowledge in mental health general curricula. Often there is a course or two taught by adjunct faculty or perhaps by a faculty member with a curiosity and interest in law who possesses some training, but not often enough are the two interrelated or integrated. Should law be recognized as a viable therapeutic tool to be used in helping the client? The question deserves discussion in depth (Barton & Sanborn, 1978; Fersch, 1980).

At a meeting with mental health professionals recently, a therapist asked a rhetorical question, "When does legal input end and meddling begin?" The message was clear. In the mind of this particular psychiatrist and perhaps other therapists as well, law and legal knowledge do not exist as part of the therapeutic process. Law is redundant. It is separate and distinct, both as a discipline and as a body of knowledge that might assist in alleviating a person's fears and anxieties. If and when a legal problem is recognized during therapy, the client is advised to see a lawyer. Therapy deals with feelings only, not the reality imposed by law (Barton & Sanborn, 1978).

There are several obvious problems inherent in the "this is a legal problem—see a lawyer" approach. One is that the lawyer may or may not know, understand, or even care about the psychological problems underlying the legal problems, nor will she/he necessarily be aware of the psychological or psychiatric history. Another is that the legal problem perceived by the therapist and the client may not be the real problem at all. If the legal and therapeutic approaches are not coordinated (Richard, 1977), seeing a lawyer might involve the client in a bitter adversary process extremely harmful to the current treatment plan. Without an interdisciplinary cooperative approach, litigation, once started, may be difficult to direct, control, or channel. Some questions would also arise concerning the difference in the therapeutic versus adversarial approach to a given problem (i.e., whether seeing a lawyer might ameliorate or exacerbate a situation). Although lawyers are also "counselors," they are not always known to be peacemakers.

It is certain that in many problem areas law has an impact that cannot be ignored (Tapp, 1976). For a therapist to guide a client through a thought process without fundamental legal knowledge is to construct a building without a solid foundation. When legal as well as psychological problems exist, they must be handled in tandem. An easing of tensions in one area may abate a crisis, but unless all legal and psychological considerations are integrated, the temporary solution is a harbinger of a more serious situation looming on the horizon.

Law and therapy go hand in hand. What are some of the obvious areas in which legal input would be essential to the therapeutic or counseling process? When should the therapist be sensitive to legal issues? What problems exist where therapy and law must co-exist? Can a therapist afford to be ignorant of the law? Can such ignorance ever be excused?

THE ELDERLY AND TERMINALLY ILL

Gerontology is emerging as an important specialty in the therapeutic process. In nursing homes and homes for the elderly, therapists are on call and on staff to counsel individuals and families through the aging process, especially as the hale and hearty become the ill and infirm.

Therapy for the aging, the dying, and the terminally ill offers a modicum of peace of mind as well as an awareness of the finite quality of life.

Additional peace of mind can also be made available through the interrelationship of the lawyer and the therapist as the therapist can encourage the clients to put their legal houses in order (Bernstein, 1979b; Bernstein, 1980). Every individual ought to have a current, valid will that disposes of his or her property in a manner commensurate with the considered wishes of the property owner. This will, together with an estate plan in a degree of complexity and sophistication commensurate with the amount of the estate and the requirements of the testator, should constantly be reviewed so that if there is a sudden change in health status, the individual who has worked a lifetime to accumulate property will be secure in the knowledge that the property disposition will be made according to his/her wishes.

Other instruments are likewise available to serve the elderly individual. These include a general or special power of attorney, a joint bank account with the right of survivorship, a two-signature bank account, a living or testamentary trust, and a myriad of banking and trust facilities available from all major banks in every city in the nation.

Also, an individual might want to make an anatomical gift as a last meaningful gesture for the good of research or to help another individual. Most states allow this gesture to be recorded on the reverse of a driver's license, whereas others proscribe certain formalities. Not everyone will want to be a donor, but at least the individual should be aware that the opportunity is available.

Many states have enacted the Natural Death Act, which permits a person to execute an instrument with certain formalities that allows the physician to refrain from using extraordinary means to keep a person alive. Usually this must be substantially supported by medical evidence, and the individual must always be medically unable to respond to treatment. Although perhaps not legally binding on physicians or surviving family, the execution of an instrument permitting a natural death may express an intention of the individual that can be honored by survivors with a clear conscience. In this instance, this suggestion alone can save thousands of dollars in unappreciated, incredibly expensive medical services. Likewise, a carefully drawn will or trust instrument can save thousands of tax dollars. It can serve as a vehicle to avoid the possibility of either a contested will or an interfamily dispute creating family differences that may never be resolved. Individuals who counsel the elderly and the infirm should consider the available legal niceties as an appropriate adjunct to the therapeutic process (Cohen, 1978).

SERVING THE SURVIVOR

Often, family therapy focuses solely on the old and infirm. The emphasis relates to the elderly individual and his or her physical and psychological needs as time slowly takes its toll. Family members and loved ones have both financial and emotional concerns which are often difficult to share openly. Potential survivors are directly involved with and interested in the estate plan of the elderly individual. Indeed, this concern may simmer slowly beneath the surface of every conversation, with each individual goaded by self-interest, but reluctant to speak because of the delicate nature surrounding family relationships (Bernstein, 1977).

Individuals often have items of real and personal property that have been sequestered unknown to other members of the family. Long before an individual's approaching disability or senility, family members should make sure that the elderly individuals have taken an inventory that accounts for all of their remaining personal and real property, which they have accumulated during their lifetime. Likewise, bank accounts may have been established years ago in hometowns and favorite banks, often for long forgotten premiums. Each year, thousands of these dollars escheat to the state, for the account owners are lost and gone forever. The potential survivor can only locate this property while the individual with knowledge of the whereabouts of each asset is alive and able to locate each item of property. These individuals should be alerted to this situation when in therapy or when consulting a chaplain or mental health professional.

In addition to a current, valid, and appropriate will, all documents of importance should be gathered together in one place and carefully inventoried. Insurance companies do not gratuitously pay death claims. They only pay when presented with a death certificate and the insurance policy or a verified copy. Insurance policies and inventories, balance sheets, stock certificates, bank books, checking accounts, and veterans benefits, as well as social security benefits, are available to survivors at the appropriate time. From a lawyer's standpoint, the family so advised can save thousands of dollars in legal fees. From the therapist's perspective, counseling survivors should be considered unethical if it is regarding merely interspousal relationships and ignoring financial realities that can cause needless grief to clients and their families, especially at a time when the world appears harsh and cruel enough.

One must keep in mind that estate litigation is always between and among surviving heirs—usually brothers, sisters, and other relatives. By careful estate planning and preparation, the potential survivors can eliminate all or most interfamily acrimonious litigation (Bernstein, 1979b).

COHABITATION

Cohabitation among single adults has been practiced for centuries. In many jurisdictions, cohabitation was not thought to have any profound or far-reaching legal consequences. Certainly no property interests were created. The Lee Marvin case (1976) indicates that single consenting adults who elect to live together, basically pooling their resources, may find personal happiness in their extramarital bliss, but at the same time they cannot escape certain specific legal consequences. When and if the union should dissolve, property as well as personal rights must be considered. The therapist who is aware of this type of living arrangement must at least make the parties aware of their potential legal involvement (DeBonis, Mercurio, Mitchelson, 1980).

Cohabiting couples should at the least create, keep, and maintain a precohabitation inventory so that should a split occur, each can leave with the same property he or she had originally. Likewise, real estate can be hopelessly entangled when two individuals feel that they have a pecuniary or proprietary interest in a piece of property, and that particular property is in the name of the other party. It is not difficult to foresee incredible inequities when property is purchased by two individuals, now cohabiting, who take the property in the name of one party or the other. The recorded owner can always sell the property and dispose of the assets. The nonrecorded owner may have an equitable claim, but enforcement in equity is a potential lawsuit with all its difficulties and ramifications. Likewise, cohabitors should review their wills and estate plans so as to accommodate the other individual in the event there is joint property.

If real or personal property is accumulated, separate lists of ownership must be established, and when nonconsumables are acquired that might be commingled, these items have to be specifically itemized for possible future distribution.

Another problem is the potential litigation that might be commenced when the cohabitors have children by a former marriage but this exotic life style is not condoned by the noncustodial spouse. Parents often take a dim view of their children living in a nonmarried household, whether heterosexual or homosexual, or in a commune, or with multiple single parents living under the same roof, or engaging in a constant series of liaisons, or even living in a sexually open marriage. Neither judges nor juries are sympathetic to cohabitation or dramatically alternative life styles. They know it exists, but it is neither fostered nor encouraged, and might easily lead to a motion to modify to change custody, filed on behalf of the noncustodial spouse. Living in sin is not a concept easily laid to rest.

One can easily envision the estate problems. Two people cohabit. Personally, they are comfortable with the arrangement. Legally, they are in jeopardy. They have given little or no thought to their wills or estate plans, children of former marriages, the potential involvement of a former spouse as guardian asserting the interest of a minor child against the surviving cohabitor's estate, nor have they considered litigation that might arise if insurance policies are not kept up.

Certain states permit a common-law marriage in which two parties live together as husband and wife and present themselves to others as if they are married. The therapist in a state that permits common-law marriage must appropriately guide a relationship that might ultimately lead to an unwanted common-law marriage. There is no such procedure as a common-law divorce. There is also no legal structure that recognizes cohabitation as a life status. The Lee Marvin case indicated that creating the relationship is somewhat easier than dissolving it. This provides a caveat to all therapists who deal with this modern-day sophisticated life style.

THE CHILD AS A WITNESS

Children, involuntarily, are regularly involved in litigation in which their own future as well as the future of others is to be decided by a judge or jury (Buxton, Dubin, & Haller, 1979). Often, in custody litigation as well as lawsuits involving adoption, termination of parental rights, criminal incest, battered children, child abuse, neglect, and other areas in which children are victims, they are the only witnesses to the illegal or negligent act that gave rise to their difficulty (Groves, 1980). Therapists often interview children in family therapy as well as individual therapy. They respond to children's needs and use their professional skills to relate to an exclusive legal concept not yet fully understood or recognized by the "helping" professional. This doctrine is what is in the "best interests of a child." Often the child is called upon to testify. Every family practice lawyer has seen an intimidated and frightened child, crying or whimpering, brought into the courtroom under the auspices of the court or of a parent, district attorney, guardian *ad litem* appointed by the court to represent the child or the best interests of the child, or other individual. Children may testify if they have the intelligence and capacity to provide facts about a case and if they feel a duty to tell the truth. It is not a matter of age; it is a matter of maturity (Benedek & Schetky, 1980).

The therapist cannot protect a child from offering this admissible evidence if the evidence is sought by a proper party to the litigation. The judge can decree whether the child's testimony is or is not admissible. If admissible as relevant and material to the litigation and the judge rules the child is sufficiently mature, the child must take the witness stand and testify as any other witness.

In this area the therapist has a special duty. Knowing that a child might be called to court, the therapist should first become familiarized with courtroom practices and procedures. He or she must then determine the child's cognitive stage of development as well as emotional stage and personality strength. The child should then be led through certain role-playing exercises so as to make him or her comfortable in court.

As a beginning, the child might visit the court and become personally acquainted with the courtroom decor. The child might also walk into the courtroom and sit on the witness chair. Various individuals might take the place of the judge, jury, parents, and attorney. The attorney might role play the questions to be asked and make the child feel comfortable in giving answers. The child must be clearly informed that what he or she says will not solely determine the court's decision. What the child says is only part of that which enables someone else, the judge or jury, to make the decision. The child should always be told that testifying does not indicate a lack of love for one parent or choosing one parent over another, but that it is only to explain facts and feelings for the purpose of allowing the judge to make the ultimate ruling. The child must become relaxed with the therapist as well as the various attorneys. The child should not ever be brought into court totally unprepared.

Therapists are often frightened by the drama of the adversary system. It takes little to imagine the frightening aspects that a courtroom appearance might have for a child. It is possible to assert that a particular child should not be a witness and that being a witness might produce long-range detrimental effects. However, this is not sufficient reason to keep a child off of the witness stand if the child is properly called for a legitimate reason by a party to the litigation. A legally competent child may be asked to testify, and the role of the therapist is to understand this potential hazard and, when the potential hazard becomes real, to acquaint the child with the task that must be performed so that it can be performed with the least damage to the child.

Preventive therapy in this area is absolutely essential: First, the rules of the game must be clearly understood. Second, the therapist and child must be prepared. Third, the therapist must be available for post-testimony trauma. Fourth, the child might need or desire a therapist, attorney, or both to serve as guardian or attorney ad litem, so as to provide the child with an advocate both of the child as well as his or her best interests (Bernstein, 1979a; Buxton, Dubin, & Haller, 1979).

THE PREMARITAL AGREEMENT

Often, religious reasons mandate that parties intending to marry seek the help of a clergyman. Other individuals, especially those marrying for the second or third time, might sensibly seek the input of a therapist to bring to the surface premarital problems and to explore the new relationship each is about to enter. In this era of the blended family, where an early marriage was entered into basically unencumbered, the second or third relationship ought to be entered into with some caution regarding legal and property rights before, during and perhaps even following the marriage should it fail. One can easily picture the typical American family of "your" children, "my" children, and possibly "our" children. Then there is your property before marriage, my property before marriage, and our property during marriage. Then, in a later marriage, there are children and grandchildren as well, often former spouses, and business or financial arrangements and obligations of various degrees of complexity. Likewise, there might also be items of inheritance from either side of the family that can cause ownership problems.

One can easily envision two parties immediately prior to marriage who have real and personal property, children, insurance, family obligations, and perhaps properties secured by substantial debts. Each wants to marry. Each is committed to the new relationship. Each is incredibly fearful of a full disclosure of feelings and finances. To bring up a premarital agreement might frighten off the other party. The therapist's failure to be a catalyst in this area, vigorously urging both parties to review their needs, expectations, and fears, is unforgivable.

As a basic minimum, each party should have an inventory. The premarital agreement can easily provide that in the event of a divorce, each party leaves the marriage with the property they brought in. In addition, the characterization, ownership, and control of property earned during the marriage may be fixed so that each party can be secure in the knowledge that the interest in his/her separate property as well as monies earned during the marriage remain personal and individual, apart from that of his/her spouse. Also, at this time, a full review of each party's insurance and estate plan must be made so that each is comforted by the knowledge that loved ones will not be isolated and that family expectations and obligations are respected.

Parties entering into a marriage in this complex era must be forewarned and then forearmed. The therapist who counsels premarital couples owes it to these clients to at least mention the possibility of the premarital agreement. Like other concepts, this might be rejected. The parties may not want to face up to the potential hazard or danger of negotiating finances at such a sensitive time. Nevertheless, the therapist who does not bring this issue to the forefront is doing a disservice to the clients. Parties who marry, worried about the security of their estate, are bound to display this insecurity with inappropriate and detrimental conduct as time goes on. Clandestine contracts, secret wills, gifts to children, trust funds, and even conveyances of property may protect heirs, but at the same time create incredible anxieties. One cannot enter into a meaningful and committed relationship hobbled by undue individual concerns over money, property, insurance, wills, and the pressures of potential heirs.

DIVORCE/FAMILY COUNSELING

A multitude of individuals seek therapists for counseling originally designed to preserve a marriage. The result of therapy is often a healthy, vibrant, exciting marriage, or at least a marriage that does not dissolve by divorce. Also, the therapy creates an awareness in either or both parties that the marriage relationship is about to terminate. Assume that the unhappy or unfulfilled marriage is about to end in a divorce. The divorce may not occur at a certain time, but, in reasonable therapeutic probability, it appears imminent.

Should this be the case, the therapist and client should be aware that the possibility of insupportability as a ground for divorce is present in every marriage. The time-honored causes such as adultery, cruelty, abandonment, and confinement in a mental institution still exist by statute, but in the vast majority of cases, divorces are granted on the grounds of insupportability, or "no fault." Thus, individuals no longer argue about who obtains the divorce. Rather, substantial arguments are made concerning custody, visitation, child support, and the division of property. The experience of most lawyers is that custody is agreed on by the parties involved, and it is only in a relatively rare instance that a bitterly contested custody battle takes place. Often, with the help of a competent therapist, the parties can arrive at a reasonable agreement concerning custody and visitation suited to geography as well as individual tastes (Adams & Solow, 1977; Howe, 1977).

Problems usually arise concerning child support and the division of property. In this area the therapist must be convinced that each party understands the financial realities of the divorce process. The noncustodial parent must know approximately what he or she is to pay the custodial parent in child support, and the custodial parent as well as the noncustodial parent must each itemize their personal budgets so as to accommodate their new life style in the best manner possible. Likewise, although judges have discretion in dividing the accumulation from a marriage, they have no crystal ball and often simply split the personal and real property down the middle. Therapists usually have little or no training in family finances. Therefore, several basic rules should apply, subject to being adapted by the judge and the jurisdiction. Child support is often a certain percentage of take-home pay; 20% for one child, 25% for two children, 28% for three children, and 30% for four children. Is this too much to pay or not enough to receive? That is an intellectual as well as a practical problem. The real dilemma is to fit these payments and receipts into a new life style.

Likewise, the parties must assemble a complete, accurate, and up-to-date inventory. Even though it might not be appropriate for the therapist to play judge and divide the assets, it would certainly be helpful to consult with an attorney who, through experience and education, can probably suggest a distribution that a court would approve and that would be fair and equitable to both parties. Through contact with an attorney, the therapist can also become aware of the differences that arise between the written word and the practical application. For example, the therapist should know that a written court order for child support does not guarantee that the custodial parent will always receive child support from the noncustodial parent. The therapist should know that child snatching, even if a felony in some states and prohibited by legal statute, nevertheless occurs, and that the emotional and financial drain in locating a snatched child is devastating. The therapist should be aware of the attitudes of police and law enforcement officers who often will not become involved in family disputes, even when a breach of the peace is involved. In summary, the therapist must not only be aware of the law itself but must also be aware of its enforcement and practical application.

Parties who receive counseling from a therapist may end up being divorced. This is a fact of life. The therapist who is knowledgeable in divorce procedures and financing can best prepare the client for a realistic postdivorce life style. The therapist may not be able to prevent the divorce, but he or she can often prevent postdivorce depression by anticipating problems that he or she is aware may arise in the future.

Custody and Courtroom Testimony

Most courts require that children involved in child custody (Fenster, Gerber, & Litwack, 1979-1980) proceedings see a court-appointed or a private therapist. The therapist may pursue additional individual counseling with the children involved, and often counsels the parents and occasionally extended family members, friends, teachers, school counselors, and neighbors. When custody is involved, the stakes are incredibly high. The court will often qualify the therapist as an expert because of his or her education, training, and experience, and the opinion of the expert is weighed heavily by the judge or jury who respect professional competence as well as sensible preferred options (Levy, 1978).

The therapist who enters the courtroom must be an advocate of his/her own professionally acquired point of view. The therapist who has interviewed a family, offered professional input, and who then arrives at a conclusion as to who is the best individual to serve as custodial parent now has acquired an additional obligation. This point of view must be clearly exhibited to the court in a manner that is meaningful and persuasive. All can easily be lost if the therapist has arrived at a correct conclusion but is unable to transmit this conclusion to the judge or jury in a way that creates meaningful and persuasive evidence.

Therapists must present their credentials clearly and impressively. They must role play the question-and-answer courtroom scenario and must offer the attorney a list of relevant questions they wish to be asked. Many a lawyer has been confronted by a therapist following the courtroom drama only to be reminded that the therapist had more to offer, but the attorney neglected to ask the right questions. Thus, all relevant questions must be prepared in advance, the questions framed in clear language, understandable to a judge or jury, and the answers available. Likewise, the therapist must be prepared for the withering cross fire of adverse cross-examination, designed to destroy, intimidate, harass, and confuse the therapist who sits in the witness chair in unfamiliar and uncomfortable surroundings. The rules of evidence that apply to therapists are universal. Therapists who become part of the forensic scene as an advocate of their point of view can only do so effectively with study and practice. The opportunity for study is available in most communities. Individuals are entitled to their day in court. The therapist owes each client a personal duty to make that day a satisfying experience. The client must leave the courtroom convinced that his/her day in court was professionally presented in the best possible manner.

There Is No Excuse

Although the therapist can blissfully offer therapy in a professional manner without any knowledge of the law, this would be unfair, inconsiderate, lazy, and unprofessional, as well as unrealistic. Feelings and attitudes must be considered in light of reality. The law offers a portion of that reality. If the therapist is not familiar with the law that affects the client's problems, the evolving attitudinal and behavioral changes will be short-lived. Unless the legal problems are faced along with the personal and psychological problems, the attitudinal changes may revert back to pretherapy days, thus recreating old problems. Family therapists must be aware of the laws that affect particular individual clients. They must recognize the law not to practice it, but to recognize problem areas and to make referrals where appropriate. They cannot make a referral if they are not aware that a legal problem exists. Ignorance of the law may be an excuse in the malpractice area in the sense that therapists are not liable for failure to offer legal advice nor would they be liable for failure to refer a client to an attorney. But, certainly, effective therapy must at least consider the options that are allowable and involve these options in the therapeutic process.

Since in most cases the therapist is in a discipline that is licensed by the state, the licensing practices and procedures must be understood (Slovenko, 1966, 1973). Every discipline has a code of ethical responsibility. Upon joining a national organization, the therapist subscribes to the ethical code, and if the ethical code is violated and a malpractice suit is commenced, the code of ethics may be introduced as evidence to determine the standard of care due and owing to clients. Deviation from the published norm may be negligence. Thus, not only must therapists be familiar with the statute and case law involved, but they must also be acquainted with the professional codes of ethics and standards of their discipline.

Although some colleges and universities offer introductory courses in law and therapy, such education is only the tip of the iceberg. Also, forensic education becomes rapidly obsolete as law continuously evolves. Continuing education is available and essential. Numerous articles and books are available: *The New Face of Legal Psychiatry* (Robitscher, 1972), *Forensic Psychiatry* (Sadoff, 1975), *Psychiatry and Law* (Slovenko, 1973), *Confidentiality in Social Work—Issues and Principles* (Wilson, 1978), and *Coping with Psychiatric and Psychological Testimony* (Ziskin, 1981). Professional journals contain countless articles that impact on the law and the helping professions. Theme journals and journals such as the *Law and Social Work Quarterly* contain educational materials. Seminars, workshops, and symposia are constantly sponsored by universities, health care and public agencies, and private organizations. An update in the literature can be obtained inexpensively from the computer data bank of the National Institute of Mental Health, *Psychological Abstracts*, the National Library of Medicine, and other professional sources.

Lawyers will speak at the mere hint of an invitation, usually well prepared and generally without charge. Law schools organize free lectures any time an audience is interested as a part of their community public relations. Ignorance of the law? There is no excuse. The information is available, free, or inexpensive, and is there for the asking.

REFERENCES

Adams, P. L., & Solow, R. A. Custody by agreement: Child psychiatrist as child advocate. *Journal of Psychiatry and Law*, 1977, 5, 77-100.

Barton, W. E., & Sanborn, C. J. *Law and the mental health professions: Friction at the interface.* New York: International Universities Press, 1978.

Benedek, E., & Schetky, D. H. *Child psychiatry and the law.* New York: Brunner/Mazel, 1980.

Bernstein, B. E. The attorney ad litem: Guardian of the rights of child and incompetents. *Social Casework*, 1979, 60, 463-470. (a)

Bernstein, B. E. Lawyer and therapist as an interdisciplinary team: Interfacing for the terminally ill. *Death Education*, 1979, 3, 11-19. (b)

Bernstein, B. E. Lawyer and therapist as an interdisciplinary team: Serving the survivors. *Death Education*, 1980, 1, 277-291.

Buxton, M., Dubin, J. D., & Haller, L. H. The use of the legal system as a mental health service for children. *Journal of Psychiatry and Law*, 1979, 7, 7-48.

Cohen, E. S. Editorial: Law and aging, lawyers and gerontologists. *The Gerontologist,* 1978, *18,* 229.

De Bonis, E. G., Mercurio, P., & Mitchelson, M. M. Pretrial considerations and trial tactics in Marvin-type litigation. *American Journal of Trial Advocacy,* 1980, *4,* 1-15.

Fenster, A., Gerber, G. L., & Litwack, T. R. The proper role of psychology in child custody disputes. *Journal of Family Law,* 1979-1980, *18,* 269-300.

Fersch, E. A., Jr. *Psychology and psychiatry in courts and corrections: Controversy and change.* New York: Wiley, 1980.

Groves, J. R. Psychologist and psychological evidence in child protection hearings. *Queens Law Journal,* 1980, *5,* 241-268.

Howe, A. W. Divorce: Critical issues for legal and mental health professionals. *Urban and Social Change Review,* 1977, *10,* 15-21.

Levy, A. M. The resolution of child custody cases: The courtroom or consultation room. *Journal of Psychiatry and Law,* 1978, *6,* 499-517.

Marvin v. Marvin, 557 P. 2d 106 (Cal. 1976). Minnesota has agreed: Carlson v. Olson, 3 F.L.R. 2467 (Minn. 1977).

Richard, B. (Ed.). *Psychiatrists and the legal process.* New York: Insight, 1977.

Robitscher, J. The new face of legal psychiatry. *American Journal of Psychiatry,* 1972, *129,* 91-97.

Sadoff, R. L. *Forensic psychiatry.* Springfield, Ill.: Charles C Thomas, 1975.

Slovenko, R. *Psychotherapy, confidentiality, and privileged communication.* Springfield, Ill.: Charles C Thomas, 1966.

Slovenko, R. *Psychiatry and law.* Boston, Mass.: Little, Brown, 1973.

Tapp, J. L. Psychology and the law: An overture. *Annual Review of Psychology,* 1976, *27,* 359-404.

Wilson, S. J. *Confidentiality in social work—issues and principles.* The Free Press, N.Y.: 1978.

Ziskin, J. *Coping with psychiatric and psychological testimony* (3rd ed.). Venice, Calif.: Law and Psychology Press, 1981.

7. Issues in Family Law: Implications for Therapists

R. Barry Ruback, J.D., Ph.D.
Department of Psychology
Georgia State University
Atlanta, Georgia

Seven

FAMILY THERAPISTS HAVE BECOME INCREASINGLY AWARE that they operate in a legal context. Statutes, regulations, and court decisions govern who can practice marriage and family therapy (Sporakowski & Staniszewski, 1980), to whom third-party payment can be made, and the standards of care in malpractice suits (Harris, 1973). In addition to knowledge of these legal issues, family therapists need to be familiar with the basic principles of family law, since they often deal with couples considering divorce and are often called upon to testify about such problems as child custody.

The family therapist may interact with the legal system in three important ways: as an expert witness, as a resource for therapy in required conciliation proceedings, and as a source of information leading to intervention by the state. In these roles, it is essential that the therapist understand the applicable law. Although practicing therapists are aware of the importance of knowing the legal ramifications of their own and their clients' actions, graduate students still, for the most part, leave school with little knowledge of family law. Clearly, some sort of legal education for therapists should be required (Derdeyn, 1975), both in graduate school and as part of a continuing education program. As Bernstein (1982) argues in an article in this collection, there is really no excuse for a practicing family therapist not to know the law relevant to families.

This article, based on a course in family law offered at Georgia State University, briefly describes the kinds of legal information that a family therapist ought to be familiar with. It must be stressed that the relevant law is too complex to be covered in depth here; for more thorough discussions of the relevant law, the reader is referred to the cited references. For problems with a specific case, the reader should see an attorney.

In terms of general references on family law, there are several that the family therapist should be acquainted with. Krause's (1977) paperback *Family Law in a Nutshell* is a readable survey of family law. A more complete summary is Clark's *The Law of Domestic Relations* (1968). The therapist should also be aware of the major legal textbooks in the area, since they can often be helpful references. These textbooks include *Cases and Materials on Family Law* by Areen (1978); *Cases and Problems on Domestic Relations* by Clark (1974); *Family Law: Cases and Materials* by Ploscowe, Foster, and Freed (1972); and *Cases on Domestic Relations* by Wadlington and Paulsen (1978). Finally, the encyclopedic book *The Family and the Law: Problems for Decision in the Family Law Process* by Goldstein and Katz (1965) contains excerpts from many sources and should prove very informative for the family therapist.

THE LEGAL PROCESS

To many family therapists, the legal system is an unknown world in which abstruse concepts and arcane language are used. Although it is not necessary that the therapist gain sufficient skill to become an attorney, he or she should have some knowledge of the legal process, including familiarity with basic legal procedure and legal research. With regard to legal procedure, it is important for the therapist to understand the basic workings of a trial court, since he or she might be called upon to explain what will happen to his or her clients in court (see Bernstein, 1982). The therapist should also be generally familiar with the way legal research is conducted because a working knowledge of case citations and legal periodicals might prove helpful to the therapist who would like to learn more about a specific case or topic in family law. Thus, therapists should know the way cases and statutes are cited and where they can be found, and should have some familiarity with the *Index to Legal Periodicals*, the major index of publications in law. For the person who is interested in learning more about legal research, there are several books on the topic, including those by Bander (1978), Cohen (1971), and Lloyd (1974). Probably the most complete is *Fundamentals of Legal Research* by Jacobstein and Mersky (1977).

HISTORY AND PRESENT CONTEXT OF FAMILY LAW

In addition to being familiar with basic legal processes, the family therapist should know something about the history of family law and the recent trends in the area. In terms of history, the therapist might want to look at the articles by Katz (1980) and Zainaldin (1980). In recent years family law has become increasingly important in both practical and theoretical realms. In practical terms, matters relating to family law have been estimated to compose more than half of all of the civil cases filed in the United States (Hennessey, 1980). In theoretical terms, family law issues have become increasingly subject to constitutional scrutiny. For example, the Supreme Court has decided such family issues as procreation, abortion, and marriage on the basis of due process and equal protection considerations (Note, 1980). Moreover, with changing life styles, particularly cohabitation without marriage, courts have increasingly adapted concepts from other areas of the law (e.g., implied contract or partnership, constructive trust) to traditional family matters (Douthwaite, 1979; Hennessey, 1980).

LAW OF MARRIAGE

Because the right to marry is "fundamental"[1] the state can significantly interfere with this right only in the presence of a "compelling state interest" (see Glendon, 1976). Thus, miscegenation statutes would be unconstitutional under this standard.[2] However, statutes prohibiting incest probably do meet this standard (Krause, 1977). Courts have held that the fundamental right to marry does not include homosexual marriages.[3]

State laws typically require the parties in a marriage to meet a certain minimum age requirement, to be of sound mind, to be tested for venereal disease, and to wait for a specified period of time (often 3 days) between the time the marriage license is issued and the time the marriage is solemnized. The two major types of marriage are ceremonial marriage, in which the marriage is performed in a ceremony before a civil or religious authority, and common law marriage, in which the parties live together as husband and wife without having participated in a marriage ceremony. For both types of marriage the parties must have the legal capacity to make a contract and must actually make an agreement to marry (Clark, 1974).

Although there can be problems in determining whether a valid marriage exists, increasingly more common are problems arising in connection with prenuptial agreements and cohabitation without marriage. Prenuptial agreements are simply contracts entered into by the parties, usually relating to the transfer and distribution of property. Courts are generally reluctant to enforce prenuptial agreements that relate to the rights of the parties in the case of divorce or to the duties of the parties during marriage (Krause, 1977). A second issue that has recently become more common is nonmarital cohabitation (Crutchfield, 1981; Weitzman, 1974). Such relationships have ramifications across a number of different areas, including employment, welfare, insurance, and tort liability (Douthwaite, 1979). In a much publicized decision, the Supreme Court of California held that a cohabiting couple could make an express contract regarding their property rights, as long as sex was not part of the consideration for the agreement.[4] It must be noted that this decision has not been universally followed.[5] (See Note, 1978.) The law relating to the rights and duties of spouses during marriage is undergoing change (see, e.g., Weitzman, 1974). These changes have affected marital property rights (Glendon, 1980), as well as the extent to which abused spouses have recourse against their marital partners (Fleming, 1979).

DISSOLUTION OF MARRIAGE

Marriages can be terminated either by annulment or divorce. Annulment is a declaration by the court that for reasons existing at the time of the marriage, the marriage is void. These reasons include insanity, bigamy, fraud, duress, incest, and not being of age (Krause, 1977). Because most marriages are terminated by divorce rather than annulment and because divorce has direct implications for family therapists, the law of divorce will be discussed in some detail.

There are over 1.1 million divorces annually, affecting a slightly larger number of children (U.S. Bureau of the Census, 1980). Traditionally, divorce required that one party be at fault. The original fault grounds of adultery and physical cruelty were later expanded to include such other grounds as habitual drunkenness, willful desertion, mental cruelty, and conviction of a felony. Since the assumption was that only the innocent party was entitled to a divorce, if it could be proved that *both* parties were at fault, neither one could receive a divorce. This reasoning, called *the doctrine of recrimination,* made a contested divorce more difficult to win. Also, based on the state's interest in protecting marriages, if the two parties engaged in collusion to obtain the divorce, traditionally, divorce would be barred.

In recent years there has been a trend away from requiring fault in divorce actions (Hennessey, 1980). In only two states, Illinois and South Dakota, is fault still necessary. The remaining states allow for some type of no-fault divorce, although traditional fault grounds may still be alleged in many of these states (Freed & Foster, 1981). This trend toward no-fault divorces began in California and continued with the promulgation of the Uniform Marriage and Divorce Act (National Conference of Commissioners, 1971). According to Section 305 of this model act, the court can grant a divorce on finding that "the marriage is irretrievably broken," a decision based on "the petitioner's reasons for seeking a dissolution of the marriage and the prospect that the parties may achieve a reconciliation" (Commentary on Section 305). At present, 17 states use this standard as the sole ground for divorce, and an additional 17 states have added irretrievable breakdown to traditional fault grounds (Freed & Foster, 1981).

Although fault is no longer required, in most states divorce is not immediately granted merely on the consent of the parties to the divorce. In most states, there must be evidence to support the finding that the marriage is irretrievably broken (Freed & Foster, 1981). Also, several states have a mandatory minimum waiting period after the action is filed before the court may grant a divorce. Furthermore, many states grant courts the discretion to require couples to undergo counseling and conciliation. The stated purpose of these barriers to automatic divorce is to avoid the hasty dissolution of marriages that might still be viable and that, but for liberalized divorce procedures, would remain intact. Because of the fundamental importance of marriage to society, requirements preventing such hasty dissolutions are probably constitutionally permissible (Note, 1980).

The requirement of conciliation conferences prior to the granting of divorce has obvious and important implications for family therapists, since often they are the ones who are called upon to conduct these conferences. For example, Iowa law gives the court the power to require the parties to participate in conciliation efforts conducted by "the domestic relations division of the court, if established, public or private marriage counselors, family service agencies, community health centers, physicians and clergymen."[6]

In many states, conciliation efforts are conducted by a court-employed counselor. It has been argued that by having such efforts connected to the court, the parties are more likely to undergo the counseling in good faith, and the court can be assured that the counselors are competent and trained to deal with families rather than individuals (Orlando, 1978). Orlando also argues that in areas in which conciliation is required, about 75% of the couples reconcile and stay together for at least a year. Furthermore, when reconciliation is not possible, the required counseling helps reduce the number of custody disputes and contested divorces. In contrast to Orlando, other individuals have questioned the value of required conciliation given the expense, low probability of success, and shortage of trained personnel (see Krause, 1977). Although there is some question about the effectiveness of mandatory conciliation efforts, such counseling is likely to continue because of the state's interest in preserving marriages.

Because most states have adopted no-fault divorce laws, problems in divorces center almost completely on matters relating to property. Thus, the therapist should be aware of the laws relating to property settlements, alimony, and child support. A property settlement is a division of all property acquired by either spouse after marriage. Alimony is support for the dependent spouse, made in periodic payments or in a lump sum. Child support is an obligation to pay the child's custodian an allowance for the support of minor children. The law regarding property settlements, alimony, and child support is summarized in Clark (1974) and Krause (1977). A common problem relating to these property issues after divorce is that the supporting spouse does not have enough income to make these payments and still support him or herself (Eisler, 1977).

ESTABLISHING THE PARENT-CHILD RELATIONSHIP

The creation of the parent-child relationship comprises four major topics: abortion, paternity, legitimacy, and adoption (Krause, 1977). Because of space limitations, paternity and legitimacy will not be discussed here. The reader is referred to Clark (1974) for a discussion of these issues. With regard to abortion, the Supreme Court in *Roe v. Wade* held that (a) during the first trimester of pregnancy, the state had no compelling interest that outweighed the mother's right to privacy; (b) during the second trimester, the state did have a compelling interest in the mother's health and therefore could reasonably regulate the abortion procedure;

and (c) during the third trimester (viability), the state had a compelling interest in protecting the life of the fetus and therefore could regulate and even prohibit abortion.[7] Since that decision, the Supreme Court has addressed the question of whether or not consent by the woman's husband or parent is required before the abortion can be performed. In *Planned Parenthood of Missouri v. Danforth*[8] the Court held that such consent was not required. More recently, questions have arisen concerning access to abortion by those who are unable to pay for it themselves.

With regard to adoption, several issues have been raised. One major question concerns the appropriate legal response to the black market of babies who are sold for adoption (e.g., Podolski, 1975). A second issue in the area of adoption is whether or not single persons can adopt children. Generally, courts prefer that children be adopted by couples, since two parents can provide a more natural environment (Krause, 1977). However, given the many problems in finding homes for some children (e.g., those who are older, handicapped, or from minority groups), more courts are allowing adoptions by single persons. A third issue in adoptions is whether or not the prospective adoptive parents are of the same religion and race as the child. Generally, courts prefer that the parents and child be from the same religious and racial groups (Simon & Altstein, 1977).

A fourth issue that has arisen in connection with adoption concerns the rights of an unmarried father (Bedwell, 1979). The Wisconsin Supreme Court in *Rothstein v. Lutheran Social Services*[9] held, on remand from the Supreme Court of the United States in light of *Stanley v. Illinois*[10] that an unwed father's consent was necessary before there could be a valid adoption. Other state courts seem to have taken similar positions (Kern, 1979). More recent Supreme Court decisions have suggested that noncustodial, irresponsible unmarried fathers may have less authority to veto an adoption than do either married fathers[11] or unmarried mothers.[12]

PARENTS' RIGHTS AND DUTIES TO CHILDREN

Parents have the right to make decisions affecting the welfare of their children as long as they do not violate the laws that protect children (Krause, 1977). Issues in this area have arisen regarding education[13] and medical care (Hirschberg, 1980). From the standpoint of the family therapist, the most important issues concern child abuse and neglect. If a court finds that a parent did abuse or neglect his or her children, it may remove the children, temporarily or permanently, from the custody of the parent. It may also "appoint a temporary or permanent guardian who may be an individual or State or private institution (such as a state department of family services) and who takes control over the child's well being" (Krause, 1977, p. 241). In some cases, the parent does not lose his or her parental rights even when a guardian is appointed. In severe cases of abuse or neglect, the state may move to terminate the parent's rights to his or her children (see Browning & Weiner, 1979; Muench & Levy, 1979), including allowing adoption of the child (Chemerinsky, 1979). In a recent decision, which might have broad ramifications, the Supreme Court of the United States held that indigent parents have no automatic right to counsel when they are threatened with the removal of their children.[14]

The policy question of when the state should become involved in parent-child relations was addressed in a recent book by Goldstein, Freud, and Solnit (1979). These authors argue that only gross failures of parental care, such as disappearance without making provisions for the child's care, conviction of a sexual offense against the child, or inflicting or attempting to inflict severe bodily injuries on the child should be grounds for state intervention. Goldstein et al. would exclude such vaguely defined terms as *unfit home* and *emotional neglect* as bases for intervention because they do not provide fair warning to parents and place little control over participants in the child placement process.

CHILD CUSTODY IN DIVORCE

In only a small percentage of contested divorces is child custody the source of the dispute (Woody, 1977), and in most divorces the parties usually agree on a custody arrangement. In about 85% of the cases, custody is awarded to the mother without contest from the father (Slovenko, 1973; Weitzman & Dixon, 1979). According to Slovenko, this tendency for fathers not to challenge the designation of the mother as custodian results from fathers' recognition that (a) the mother can often give the children better care, (b) the children often want to be with the mother, and (c) the courts are likely to award custody of the children to the mother anyway (Foster & Freed, 1980).

This last reason, the tendency for courts to award custody to the mother, is the result of a presumption termed the *tender years* doctrine. According to this doctrine, until nearing the period of adolescence, a child is presumed to benefit most from being in the custody of the mother (but see Orthner & Lewis, 1979). This general preference for the mother in child custody cases came into existence in the middle of the 19th century, following a long period in which it was believed that the father was better able to care for the child (Weiss, 1979). In the period following the Civil War, custody of children in their tender years was routinely awarded to the mother unless the mother was judged to be unfit. Once the children were past their tender years, the presumption was that the father would be given custody of the boys and the mother would be given custody of the girls, although courts were reluctant to separate siblings (Krause, 1977).

Since the early 1970s, the tender years doctrine has been rejected by legislative action or court decision in 37 states (Freed & Foster, 1981) and has given way to the notion that custody should be awarded on the basis of what is in the best interests of the child. According to Section 402 of the Uniform Marriage and Divorce Act (National Conference of Commissioners, 1971):

> The court shall determine custody in accordance with the best interests of the child. The court shall consider all relevant factors including: (1) the wishes of the child's parent or parents as to his custody; (2) the wishes of the child as to his custodian; (3) the interaction and interrelationship of the child with his parents, his siblings, and any other person who may significantly affect the child's best interests; (4) the child's adjustment to his home, school, and community; and (5) the mental and physical health of all individuals involved. The court shall not consider conduct of a proposed custodian that does not affect his relationship to the child (p. 241).

According to the commentary on this section, the judge may also rely on traditional presumptions (e.g., preference to a parent over a nonparent, preference to the custodian agreed upon by the parties) as long as the decision is made in the best interests of the child.

Although the standards of the best interests test appear to be clearly defined, there can be several problems in its application (Brosky & Alford, 1977). First, with regard to the wishes of the child, which are to be considered as a factor in 18 states and are controlling in Georgia, if the child is 14 years or older and the parents are not judged unfit (Freed & Foster, 1981), the child may not want to express his or her wishes out of fear of offending the nonchosen parent. Also the preferred parent may not necessarily be the one with whom the child would be better off (Weiss, 1979). Second, many of the factors depend on judges' subjective assessments of the quality of the child's interactions and adjustments and the weights that should be attached to each. Third, the best interests test asks judges to ignore conduct of the custodian that would be irrelevant to the welfare of the child. However, several authors have suggested that circumstances that could be considered to be indicative of fault in causing the breakup of the marriage could also be a sign of being an unfit parent. These behaviors would include serious emotional problems, habitual drunkenness, adultery, and gross immorality (e.g., cohabitation without marriage; Weiss, 1979).

It should be clear that the awarding of child custody on the basis of the child's best interests is not an easy decision. This decision becomes even harder when state statutes list a number of factors that the judge should consider in his or her decision, since the factors are still largely subjective and no guidance is given regarding the weight that should be attached to the various factors.

Given this state of uncertainty, judges are likely to rely on the advice of experts (Litwack, Gerber, & Fenster, 1980). If, for instance, experts will testify that the child's emotional needs can best be met by one parent over the other, that parent will usually have a strong case. Generally, the more objective these experts are, the stronger the case for the parent (Kazen, 1977). And, according to Kazen, testimony from experts regarding the emotional needs of the child is generally superior to the expressed wishes of the child.

Often, a family therapist is hired by one of the divorcing parties to testify that the interests of the child would best be served by the spouse who hired the therapist. In contrast to this procedure, it has been suggested that a mental health professional should be appointed by the court to advocate the child's interests and to serve as a consultant to the court on child development (Derdeyn, 1975), much like a court-appointed legal representative (Bersoff, 1976). In this role, the consultant could "account for the child's psychological development, the nature of children's relationship with competing parents, and medical or emotional problems of both parents and children" (Henning, 1976, p. 52).

Several states have provided court-employed personnel to conduct child-custody investigations to aid the court in its decision (Gozansky, 1976). In most states that provide such personnel, the investigator's report is available to all parties and their counsel, and the investigator can be questioned about his or her findings and recommendations. The use of investigators with specialized training is an admission by the court that it is in need of expert help in awarding custody in the best interests of the child. This trend toward increased reliance on mental health professionals in child custody decisions is likely to continue, although there is no unanimous agreement about the usefulness of psychology in child custody cases (Litwack et al., 1980; Okpaku, 1976).

In contrast to the laws of most states that grant custody to one parent and visitation rights to the other parent, there are two additional strikingly different approaches. The approach taken by Goldstein, Freud, and Solnit (1973) is that custody ought to be granted to one parent only and that this parent should determine if and when visitation by the noncustodial parent should occur. The underlying presumption of the Goldstein et al. view is that continued contact with the noncustodial parent may hinder the child's development. This view appears inconsistent with several studies (e.g., Kelly & Wallerstein, 1977; Rosen, 1977), which suggest that in many cases the child desires and needs a continued relationship with the noncustodial parent.

A second approach to the problem of custody on divorce has been joint custody of the child (Folberg & Graham, 1979; Franklin & Hibbs, 1980; Miller, 1979; Roman & Haddad, 1978; Trombetta, 1981). Eleven states now permit the court to provide for joint custody (Freed & Foster, 1981), including California, which has a presumption that joint custody should be awarded as being in the best interests of the child in cases in which the parents have agreed to joint custody. Joint custody assumes "that the aims of custody adjudication should include achieving, as far as possible, the protection of the child's relationships with both parents, easy access to both parents, and the fostering of a relationship between parents in which each is supportive of the other's parental efforts" (Weiss, 1979, p. 335). Anecdotal evidence suggests that joint custody can be effective, but this success may result from the fact that the couples using it are all self-selected. Weiss (1979) suggests that a provision for mediation or arbitration in the joint custody agreement would be helpful in preventing deadlocks over issues concerning the child (see also Franklin & Hibbs, 1980).

The family therapist needs to be aware that child custody, like alimony and child support, is not always resolved with finality (Orlando, 1978). After a decree of divorce, there may be continuing attempts to modify alimony or child support payments. Child custody may be relitigated if one spouse believes that circumstances have so changed that in the best interests of the child, custody should be modified. Even if child custody is not relitigated, there are likely to be disagreements over the care and control of the child. There may also be problems of interstate custody if the parents no longer live in the same state (Bodenheimer, 1981). The major implication of the fact that family issues can continue over a long period of time is that the family therapist may be called upon many times with regard to the problems of one family.

JUVENILE JUSTICE

Although not strictly within the domain of family law, laws relating to juvenile justice are included here because action taken against a juvenile is often based on and significantly affects the youth's family. Courts handling juveniles deal with two basic types of cases. One type, delinquency hearings, deals with juveniles who are accused of committing crimes. Prior to 1967, courts granted accused delinquents virtually none of the rights accorded to accused adult criminal offenders because the courts were said to be acting in the best interest of the youth under the *parens patriae* power of the state, which assumes that the government is responsible for the custody and control of children (Fox, 1977). In its 1967 decision *In re Gault,*[15] the Supreme Court held that a juvenile had the rights to (a) notice of charges, (b) assistance of counsel, (c) the opportunity to cross-examine witnesses, and (d) the privilege against self-incrimination. Since *Gault,* the Supreme Court has also held that a finding of delinquency for having committed a criminal act must be established by proof beyond a reasonable doubt[16] although the Court did not extend the right to trial by jury to juvenile court proceedings.[17] For summaries of the law in this area, see Feld (1981), Fox (1977), and Flicker (1979).

The second type of case regarding juveniles concerns what are called *status offenses.* They include truancy, running away, and ungovernability and are governed by laws relating to persons, minors, children, or juveniles in need of supervision. These laws have been criticized because the discretion granted judges in these cases is very broad (Glaser, 1979) and because girls seem to be treated worse than boys. For example, sexual promiscuity can be the basis for a ruling that a girl is in need of supervision, but only rarely would it be the basis of such a judgment for a boy.

ROLE OF THE FAMILY THERAPIST IN LEGAL PROCEEDINGS

As mentioned earlier, the family therapist may interact with the legal system in three important ways: as an expert witness, as a resource for therapy in required conciliation proceedings, and as a source of information leading to intervention by the state. It must be stressed that the family therapist must act within these defined roles and should never attempt to act as an attorney.

As an expert witness, the family therapist may be called upon to testify in child custody, adoption, and divorce proceedings. Several authors have offered advice to the mental health professional who will testify in court as an expert witness (e.g., Brodsky, 1977; Brodsky & Robey, 1973; Nichols, 1980; Ziskin, 1975). Basically, they emphasize the importance of adequate preparation in terms of knowing (a) the facts of the particular case and (b) the most recent theoretical and empirical evidence and critiques. These authors also point out several ploys that attorneys may use to discredit the expertise and credibility of the expert witness (e.g., "How much are you being paid for your testimony?"). As a resource for therapy, family therapists may be called upon by the court to attempt a reconciliation between spouses contemplating divorce or, failing a reconciliation, reducing the acrimony that often accompanies a divorce. This role has been discussed in an earlier section.

As a source of information, the family therapist may report instances of criminal behavior (e.g., incest, child abuse, or drug addiction) to the appropriate authorities. In many states, psychologists and social workers are required by law to report cases of suspected child abuse (Sussman, 1975). These two groups, as well as others, were added to the original group, physicians, to make salient the moral duty that all citizens have to aid defenseless children and to detect cases of abuse before the harm becomes so great as to require the services of a physician (Gulley, 1977). Most of the reporting statutes provide immunity from civil suits for reporting made in good faith, and some impose penalties for failure to report suspected cases.

These statutory requirements can pose practical and ethical problems for therapists who learn of abusive behavior during therapy. Often, therapists fail to report this behavior because they (a) do not trust any intervention by the state, since the intervention would probably be antitherapeutic; (b) do not consider the problem to be serious enough to warrant intervention by the state; or (c) do not think the problem will continue, since the family is currently in treatment (Conte, 1980). In addition, therapists may be reluctant to notify the authorities about the behavior of their clients because of their duty to maintain the confidentiality of privileged information given during therapy, although many of the reporting laws have specifically canceled such privileges (Krause, 1977). Furthermore, the case of *Tarasoff v. Regents of the University of California*[18] indicates that a conflict between confidentiality to a patient and protection of a potential victim of the patient must be resolved in favor of the potential victim. Analogous reasoning would suggest that the therapist must report instances of child abuse to protect the child, even if such reporting violates confidentiality (Dickens, 1978).

However, family therapists who become aware of child abuse through treatment of drug or alcohol abusers in family therapy should know of the possible risk of reporting these abusive acts to the appropriate authorities. Recent federal statutes and regulations greatly limit the extent to which therapists may disclose information about patients covered in the regulations. These statutes and regulations, which were intended to protect the privacy of patients and thus remove one source of reluctance to enter treatment, provide for substantial penalties for violations. Even though the regulations provide for disclosure of information to "qualified service organizations," the family therapist should not report the information to law enforcement or other authorities without first obtaining expert legal advice (Rinella & Goldstein, 1980).

IMPLICATIONS FOR THE FAMILY THERAPIST

Family law is changing rapidly as life styles change and the law attempts to deal with new circumstances. Part of this change is an increasing realization by attorneys and judges that problems in families are often more likely to be appropriately within the province of mental health rather than law. Thus, it is not surprising that legal professionals are turning more often to family therapists for help in dealing with such issues as avoiding hasty divorces and granting custody in the best interests of the child.

As is evident from this article, family law encompasses a number of different topics, all of which the therapist should have some familiarity with. Ideally, this knowledge should come from formal classroom education, supervised practical experience, and continuing education workshops. It is important that therapists have some formal education in family law while still in graduate school. In conjunction with this formal course (or courses), the student should also gain some supervised practical experience in working with families who are involved with the legal system. This experience might include working with a professional therapist who consults on child custody and adoption proceedings. Finally, it is important that the therapist have some sort of continuing education in family law, so as to keep abreast of recent changes in the law, both through statute and court decision. This continuing education can probably best be obtained through continuing education workshops. In addition, the therapist might consider looking through the two major family law journals, *Family Law Quarterly,* published by the American Bar Association, and the *Journal of Family Law,* published by the University of Louisville School of Law. To be even more current, the therapist might want to look at the *Family Law Reporter,* a loose-leaf published weekly by the Bureau of National Affairs.

In sum, given the extent to which the law governs families, particularly those who are likely to be in family therapy, therapists are doing a disservice to their clients if they are not aware of basic family law.

NOTES

[1] Zablocki v. Redhail, 434 U.S. 374 (1978).
[2] Loving v. Virginia, 388 U.S. 1 (1967).
[3] Baker v. Nelson, 291 Minn. 310, 191 N.W.2d 185 (1971).
[4] Marvin v. Marvin, 18 Cal.3d 660, 134 Cal. Rptr. 815, 557 P. 2d 106 (1976).
[5] Rehak v. Mathis, 239 Ga. 541, 238 S.E. 2d 81 (1977).
[6] Iowa Code Ann. §598.16.
[7] Roe v. Wade, 410 U.S. 113 (1973).
[8] Planned Parenthood of Missouri v. Danforth, 428 U.S. 52 (1976).
[9] Rothstein v. Lutheran Social Services, 59 Wis.2d 1, 207 N.W. 2d 826 (1973).
[10] Stanley v. Illinois, 406 U.S. 645 (1972).
[11] Quilloin v. Walcott, 434 U.S. 246 (1978).
[12] Caban v. Mohammed, 441 U.S. 380 (1979).
[13] Wisconsin v. Yoder, 406 U.S. 205 (1972).
[14] Lassiter v. Department of Social Services of Durham County, 101 S.Ct. 2153 (1981).

[15] *In re* Gault, 387 U.S. 1 (1967).
[16] *In re* Winship, 397 U.S. 358 (1970).
[17] McKeiver v. Pennsylvania, 403 U.S. 528 (1971).
[18] Tarasoff v. Regents of the University of California, 551 P.2d 334 (1976).

REFERENCES

Areen, J. *Cases and materials on family law*. Mineola, N.Y.: Foundation Press, 1978.

Bander, E.J. *Legal research and education abridgement*. Cambridge, Mass.: Ballinger, 1978.

Bedwell, M.A. The rights of fathers of non-marital children to custody, visitation and to consent to adoption. *University of California, Davis Law Review*, 1979, *12*, 412-451.

Bernstein, B.E. Ignorance of the law is no excuse: Does this apply to family therapists? In L. L'Abate (Ed.), *The Family Therapy Collections* (Vol. 1). Rockville, Md.: Aspen Systems, 1982.

Bersoff, D.N. Representation for children in custody decisions: All that glitters is not Gault. *Journal of Family Law*, 1976, *15*, 27-49.

Bodenheimer, B.M. Interstate custody: Initial jurisdiction and continuing jurisdiction under the UCCJA. *Family Law Quarterly*, 1981, *14*, 203-227.

Brodsky, S.L. The mental health professional on the witness stand: A survival guide. In B.D. Sales (Ed.), *Psychology in the legal process*. New York: Spectrum, 1977.

Brodsky, S.L., & Robey, A. On becoming an expert witness: Issues of orientation and effectiveness. *Professional Psychology*, 1973, *3*, 173-176.

Brosky, J.G., & Alford, J.G. Sharpening Solomon's sword: Current considerations in child custody cases. *Dickinson Law Review*, 1977, *81*, 683-731.

Browning, C.M., & Weiner, M.L. The right to family integrity: A substantive due process approach to state removal and termination proceedings. *Georgetown Law Journal*, 1979, *68*, 213-248.

Chemerinsky, E. Defining the "best interests": Constitutional protections in involuntary adoptions. *Journal of Family Law*, 1979, *18*, 79-113.

Clark, H.H., Jr. *Cases and problems on domestic relations*. St. Paul, Minn.: West, 1974.

Clark, H.H., Jr. *The law of domestic relations*. St. Paul, Minn.: West, 1968.

Cohen, M.L. *Legal research in a nutshell* (2nd ed.). St. Paul, Minn.: West, 1971.

Conte, J.R. *A child welfare perspective on children's versus parent's rights in incestuous families*. Paper presented at the meeting of the American Psychological Association, Montreal, September 1980.

Crutchfield, C.F. Nonmarital relationships and their impact on the institution of marriage and the traditional family structure. *Journal of Family Law*, 1981, *19*, 247-261.

Derdeyn, A. Child custody consultation. *American Journal of Orthopsychiatry*, 1975, *45*, 791-801.

Dickens, B.M. Legal responses to child abuse. *Family Law Quarterly*, 1978, *12*, 1-36.

Douthwaite, G. *Unmarried couples and the law*. Indianapolis: Smith, 1979.

Eisler, R.T. *Dissolution: No-fault divorce, marriage, and the future of women*. New York: McGraw-Hill, 1977.

Feld, B.C. Juvenile court legislative reform and the serious young offender: Dismantling the "rehabilitative ideal." *Minnesota Law Review*, 1981, *65*, 167-242.

Fleming, J.B. *Stopping wife abuse: A guide to the emotional, psychological, and legal implications for the abused woman and those helping her.* Garden City, N.Y.: Anchor Press, 1979.

Flicker, B. Discretionary law for juveniles. In L.E. Abt & I.R. Stuart (Eds.), *Social psychology and discretionary law.* New York: Van Nostrand Reinhold, 1979.

Folberg, H.J., & Graham, M. Joint custody of children following divorce. *University of California, Davis Law Review,* 1979, *12,* 523-581.

Foster, H.H., & Freed, D.J. Joint custody: Legislative reform. *Trial,* June 1980, pp. 22-27, 62.

Fox, S.J. *The law of juvenile courts in a nutshell* (2nd ed.). St. Paul, Minn.: West, 1977.

Franklin, R.L., & Hibbs, B. Child custody in transition. *Journal of Marital and Family Therapy,* 1980, *6,* 285-292.

Freed, D.J., & Foster, H.H., Jr. Divorce in the fifty states: An overview. *Family Law Quarterly,* 1981, *14,* 229-284.

Glaser, G. Discretion in juvenile justice. In L.E. Abt & I.R. Stuart (Eds.), *Social psychology and discretionary law.* New York: Van Nostrand Reinhold, 1979.

Glendon, M.A. Marriage and the state: The washing away of marriage. *Virginia Law Review,* 1976, *62,* 663-720.

Glendon, M.A. Modern marriage law and its underlying assumptions: The new marriage and the new property. *Family Law Quarterly,* 1980, *13,* 441-460.

Goldstein, J., Freud, A., & Solnit, A.J. *Beyond the best interests of the child.* New York: Free Press, 1973.

Goldstein, J., Freud, A., & Solnit, A.J. *Before the best interests of the child.* New York: Free Press, 1979.

Goldstein, J., & Katz, J. *The family and the law: Problems for decision in the family law process.* New York: Free Press, 1965.

Gozansky, N. Court-ordered investigations in child custody cases. *Willamette Law Journal,* 1976, *12,* 511-526.

Gulley, K.G. The Washington child abuse amendments. *Gonzaga Law Review,* 1977, *12,* 468-491.

Harris, M. Tort liability of the psychotherapist. *University of San Francisco Law Review,* 1973, *8,* 405-436.

Hennessey, E.F. Explosion in family law litigation: Challenges and opportunities for the bar. *Family Law Quarterly,* 1980, *14,* 187-201.

Henning, J.S. Child advocacy in adoption and divorce cases: Where is the wisdom of Solomon when we really need it? *Journal of Clinical Child Psychology,* 1976, *6,* 50-53.

Hirschberg, B.A. Who speaks for the child and what are his rights? A proposed standard for evaluation. *Law and Human Behavior,* 1980, *4,* 217-236.

Jacobstein, J.M., & Mersky, R.M. *Fundamentals of legal research.* Mineola, N.Y.: Foundation Press, 1977.

Katz, S.N. Legal history and family history: The child, the family, and the state. *Boston College Law Review,* 1980, *21,* 1025-1036.

Kazen, B.A. *When father wants custody: A lawyer's view.* Austin: State Bar of Texas, 1977.

Kelly, J.B., & Wallerstein, J.S. Part-time parent, part-time child: Visiting after divorce. *Journal of Clinical Child Psychology,* 1977, *6,* 51-54.

Kern, M.N. Unwed fathers: An analytical survey of their parental rights and obligations. *Washington University Law Quarterly,* 1979, 1029-1062.

Krause, H.D. *Family law in a nutshell.* St. Paul, Minn.: West, 1977.
Litwack, T.R., Gerber, G.L., & Fenster, C.A. The proper role of psychology in child custody disputes. *Journal of Family Law,* 1980, *18,* 269-300.
Lloyd, D. *Finding the law: A guide to legal research.* Dobbs Ferry, N.Y.: Oceana Publications, 1974.
Miller, D.J. Joint custody. *Family Law Quarterly,* 1979, *13,* 345-412.
Muench, J.H., & Levy, M.R. Psychological parentage: A natural right. *Family Law Quarterly,* 1979, *13,* 129-181.
National Conference of Commissioners on Uniform State Laws Uniform Marriage and Divorce Act. *Family Law Quarterly,* 1971, *5,* 205-251.
Nichols, J.F. The marital/family therapist as an expert witness: Some thoughts and suggestions. *Journal of Marital and Family Therapy,* 1980, *6,* 293-299.
Note, A party to a meretricious relationship is not entitled to possession of the house in which the couple meretriciously (sic) cohabited and on which she made substantial payments nor may she recover the value of her services rendered during cohabitation, because such payments and services are part of a contract based on illegal and immoral consideration. *Georgia Law Review,* 1978, *12,* 361-371.
Note, Developments in the law—the Constitution and the family. *Harvard Law Review,* 1980, *93,* 1156-1383.
Okpaku, S.R. Psychology: Impediment or aid in child custody cases. *Rutgers Law Review,* 1976, *29,* 1117-1153.
Orlando, F.A. Conciliation programs: Their effect on marriage and family life. *Florida Bar Journal,* 1978, *52,* 218-221.
Orthner, D.K., & Lewis, K. Evidence of single-father competence in childrearing. *Family Law Quarterly,* 1979, *13,* 27-47.
Ploscowe, M., Foster, H.H., Jr., & Freed, D.J. *Family law: Cases and materials.* Boston: Little, Brown, 1972.
Podolski, A.L. Abolishing baby buying: Limiting independent adoption placement. *Family Law Quarterly,* 1975, *9,* 547-554.
Rinella, V.J., & Goldstein, M.R. Family therapy with substance abusers: Legal considerations regarding confidentiality. *Journal of Marital and Family Therapy,* 1980, *6,* 319-326.
Roman, M., & Haddad, W. *The disposable parent: The case for joint custody.* New York: Holt, Rinehart & Winston, 1978.
Rosen, R. Children of divorce: What they feel about access and other aspects of the divorce experience. *Journal of Clinical Child Psychology,* 1977, *6,* 24-27.
Simon, R.J., & Altstein, H. *Transracial adoption.* New York: Wiley, 1977.
Slovenko, R. *Psychiatry and law.* Boston: Little, Brown, 1973.
Sporakowski, M.J., & Staniszewski, W.P. The regulation of marriage and family therapy: An update. *Journal of Marital and Family Therapy,* 1980, *6,* 335-348.
Sussman, A. Child abuse reporting: A review of the literature. In A. Sussman & S.J. Cohen (Eds.), *Reporting child abuse and neglect: Guidelines for legislation.* Cambridge, Mass.: Ballinger, 1975.
Trombetta, D. Joint custody: Recent research and overloaded courtrooms inspire new solutions to custody disputes. *Journal of Family Law,* 1981, *19,* 213-234.
U.S. Bureau of the Census. *Statistical Abstract of the United States: 1980* (101st ed.). Washington, D.C.: Government Printing Office, 1980.

Wadlington, W., & Paulsen, M.G. *Cases on domestic relations* (3rd ed.). Mineola, N.Y.: Foundation Press, 1978.

Weiss, R.S. Issues in the adjudication of custody when parents separate. In G. Levinger & O.C. Moles (Eds.), *Divorce and separation.* New York: Basic Books, 1979.

Weitzman, L.J. Legal regulation of marriage: Tradition and change. *California Law Review,* 1974, *62,* 1169-1277.

Weitzman, L.J., & Dixon, R.B. Child custody awards: Legal standards and empirical patterns for child custody, support and visitation after divorce. *University of California, Davis Law Review,* 1979, *12,* 473-521.

Woody, R.H. Psychologists in child custody. In B.D. Sales (Ed.), *Psychology in the legal process.* New York: Spectrum, 1977.

Zainaldin, J.S. The emergence of a modern American family law: Child custody, adoption, and the courts, 1796-1851. *Northwestern University Law Review,* 1980, *73,* 1038-1089.

Ziskin, J. *Coping with psychiatric and psychological testimony* (2nd ed.). Beverly Hills, Calif.: Law and Psychology Press, 1975.

8. The Regulation of Marital and Family Therapy

Michael Sporakowski, Ph.D.
Virginia Polytechnic Institute and State University
Blacksburg, Virginia

Eight

THE STATE REGULATION OF MENTAL-HEALTH-RELATED professions in general and marital and family therapy in particular has been of major concern to both professionals and the citizenry for at least the past two decades. Gross (1978) suggested that the "helping professions" were attempting to gain legal stature for their independent practice, approval from third-party payers (insurance) and status similar to the legal and medical professions. From a consumer's point of view, the statement has been made that regulation would ensure quality control and minimize the quackery that has from time to time existed in the provision of mental-health-related services.

Opinions vary, but based on existing state laws it is apparent that several factors have been instrumental in the development and continuance of licensing and certification. First, what are legitimate credentials for practice? Does the professional possess appropriate education and training from legitimate sources that qualify him/her for autonomous practice? Are specific guidelines available for what it is that prepares an individual to practice marital and family therapy? Do programs for such education and training exist that are reputable and carry positive educational sanction? Even though credentials may not be equal to competency (Gross, 1978; Olsen, 1978), one of the better assessments available as an indicator of professional ability is training.

Second, are there ethical standards on which the professional will base practice? Do they reflect commonly held personal, social, and professional values? Matters of personal–professional relationships and confidentiality of material discussed are major issues here. Is it the duty of the profession or the state to observe and uphold these values and ethics as a responsible member of the larger community in whom trust has been invested? As such, are certain rights and privileges as well as responsibilities accorded the professional and the clientele?

Third, is there a need for control of the professional's practice? What boundary lines delineate the practice? Who can legitimately practice and under what conditions? What interprofessional territoriality needs to be dealt with? What administrative authority needs to be exercised to be sure practice falls within prescribed limits? Do continuing professional training and education need to be encouraged? Nine states have responded to those questions affirmatively regarding marital and family therapy.

REGULATION OF MARITAL AND FAMILY THERAPY (MFT)

Legislation specifically covering the practice of MFT* currently exists in California (1963), Florida (1981), Georgia (1976), Michigan (1966), Nevada (1973), New Jersey (1969), North Carolina (1979), Utah (1973), and Virginia (1978), with Georgia's legislation in a technical state of suspension (Rutledge, 1973; Sporakowski & Staniszewski, 1980). Several other states, including Alabama, Arkansas, and Texas, regulate professional counselors but do not specifically license or certify persons in marital and family therapy, although persons living in those jurisdictions have indicated in personal correspondence that regulation *may* cover their marital and family therapy practices. Obviously a number of jurisdictions have seen sufficient need to establish a regulatory process that has become law. In addition, at least 10 other states have recently (within the past 2 years) considered MFT legislation, and 6 others have done the same prior to the 2-year period. Nevertheless, 50% of the states did not appear to be moving toward MFT regulation (Sporakowski & Staniszewski, 1980).

The lack of legislation in other states is probably related to the issue of the emergence of marital and family therapy as a distinct profession.

---

*For purposes of this article the term *marital and family therapy* is used to cover the many variations of interpersonal treatment that focus on marriages and families. The terminology varies by jurisdiction. North Carolina and Florida are the only states that use therapy/therapist. California refers to marriage, family and child counselors. Michigan's 1974 act was specific to marriage counseling.

Although support from the various mental-health-related professions has varied, generally speaking professional organizations representing psychology, social work, and medicine, and the diverse group included in the American Personnel and Guidance Association have been resistant to the anticipated intrusion of such legislation into their professional domains. In the July/August 1981 issue of *The California Therapist,* this resistance is once again discussed: "The psychiatrists and psychologists have asserted that we do not [do] therapy—we only 'give advice'—so we should be called counselors, not therapists" (cover page). At the individual level, even though few clinical psychologists have received any training in MFT, many, if not most, feel they are qualified to do such treatment. Therefore, regulation beyond what their license already covers seems nonessential. In California this recently became an issue when a psychologist who wanted to advertise MFT as a service he provided was told by the regulatory board that he would need the appropriate license. Current legislative efforts seem to be at a relative standstill because of the professional boundary maintenance impasses and the "sunset review" stances taken by many legislatures that seem to result in an attitude of "no new legislation is good legislation."

No one model regulatory code for MFT has been enacted in all states, even though the American Association for Marriage and Family Therapy has one available (Nichols, 1974). It would appear that this is as much a result of a states rights attitude in legislatures as it is an attempt by individual states to meet the needs of their citizens. The resulting hodgepodge of specifically regulated issues varies greatly, as do the assumptions and definitions on which they are based. For example, three states certify (restrict title usage), and six license (specify function as well as title); a doctoral degree is required of most professionals in Michigan and New Jersey, whereas the master's degree is generally sufficient in the others; postgraduate experience runs from 1 to 5 years minimum; three states set minimum age requirements; and, supervised experience, post-degree, may not be specifically required or be for as long as 2 years. (Additional specific details may be found in Sporakowski & Staniszewski, 1980.)

SIGNIFICANCE TO THE PRACTITIONER

A number of issues related to regulation have potential importance for the marital and family therapy practitioner.

What and Who Is Covered?

Generally, the boundaries of practice are negatively defined using exclusions or exemptions from licensure/certification. Persons practicing within the guidelines of another professional license are typically excluded as long as the individual does not claim practice as an MFT. What this most often means is that someone holding another appropriate license (e.g., psychologist, social worker) could deal with treatment of marital problems but not advertise as an MFT. California has been specific about this as previously noted.

Other exemptions frequently include persons employed by governmental agencies, schools, and colleges; clergy, when performing duties normally as part of their pastoral responsibilities; employees of non-profit or charitable agencies where the practice is performed solely under the supervision of those agencies; students or "interns" in a training status; and individuals practicing under the supervision of a licensed MFT with state approval. Specific information is summarized in Sporakowski & Staniszewski (1980) and is spelled out in detail in each state's legislation. Interpretation of these regulations is generally left up to the governing agency and ultimately the courts, although many persons would feel it is primarily an ethical, professional matter.

Academic Experience and Qualifications

To qualify for licensing or certification the individual must possess a minimum of a master's degree in social work, marriage, family and child counseling, or the behavioral sciences, including but not limited to sociology, psychology, pastoral counseling, or psychiatric nursing. Two states go significantly beyond that minimum: (a) New Jersey will accept only one master's degree, social work, or a doctorate in appropriate fields, and (b) Michigan requires a doctorate unless the master's degree is in social work, marriage, or pastoral counseling. Virginia's specialty designation in marriage and family counseling requires a master's degree of at least 60 semester hours (considerably more than an average length master's) and spells out four specific areas of coursework in which a minimum of 15 semester hours must be taken: dynamics of marriage and family systems; human sexuality; marriage and family counseling theory and techniques; and supervised practicum in marriage and family counseling.

Experience qualifications vary from Nevada's 1 year of postgraduate experience in marriage and family counseling to New Jersey's 5 years of full-time counseling experience, at least 2 of which must have been in marriage counseling. California, Georgia, Michigan, New Jersey, Utah, and Virginia require that at least some of that experience be under supervision, preferably by someone qualified in the specialty area. Generally, this has been quite possible in metropolitan areas but less likely for those desiring to practice in rural areas unless they were willing to travel some distance to meet with a supervisor. The latter situation has also been potentially problematic for some persons wishing to obtain clinical membership in organizations as the American Association for Marriage and Family Therapy where no approved supervisors may have been within reasonable driving range. Often alternative plans have been arranged at the discretion of the governing boards and agencies. Only Virginia has set up specific qualifications for designated supervisors.

The Licensure/Certification Process

In addition to the basic application, academic credentials, letters of reference, and documents on practice, six states require either written or oral examinations. In Virginia the applicant must pass the written and oral examinations for the generic license as a professional counselor and then the specialty designation examinations for marriage and family counselor. A work sample based on a case counseled must also be presented.

Application-processing fees, examination fees, and certificate fees vary considerably. Application fees range from $15 to $50. Examination fees vary from $30 to $75. License/certificate fees range from $15 to $75 with renewals varying from $15 to $75, some covering up to 2 years. Each jurisdiction has its own fee structure.

Licensure/certification may be suspended or revoked for a variety of reasons and is typically seen as a misdemeanor with fines up to $500 possible. Most frequent violations include fraud or deceit practiced on the governing board, conviction of crimes, violation of client confidentiality, unethical or professional behavior, and misuse of narcotics. Generally the specifics of these violations are well defined within the code itself. Identification of violations is seen as a responsibility of those persons licensed or certified (as per the ethical standards outlined in the various codes), as well as the general public. Usually a "friendly remonstrance" is seen as ethically sufficient unless violations are repeated or blatant and involved with criminal acts.

A BROADER PERSPECTIVE

The concept of regulation is not a new one. Many opinions are in evidence in the professional literature as to the usefulness of regulation, both for the public and for the profession. Gross (1978), in reviewing the state of licensing across several professions, concluded that the evidence reveals licensing to be a mystifying arrangement that promises protection of the public but that actually institutionalizes a lack of accountability to the public (p. 1009). He also attacked the linkage assumed to be in existence between licensing and quality/competence, finding, among other things, that 38 of 50 states licensing physicians do not specify professional incompetence as a reason for disciplinary action. His final conclusion was that licensing regulations are not providing a structure in which effective solutions to health care and helping services problems can be found.

The expansion of licensure coverage to professionals other than those traditionally regulated is another issue of importance. More specifically, Forster (1978) sees that counseling has evolved under a "protective wing" from psychology and that specialization in the form of marriage and family counseling has attained recognition at a national level in the form of accreditation. Whether to regulate comprehensively (i.e., as counselor generalists) or to go the specialty route (i.e., MFTs) is open for debate and not an issue on which consensus is currently found. One stance taken is that for MFT to achieve professional creditability it must have its own set of licensing and certification laws. It is this author's opinion that a more general approach, for example a Board of Behavorial Science Examiners, wherein the several distinct professions and specialties are jointly covered, offers greater potential for both the professional and the client. Piecemeal legislative efforts of the past have done little more than to slice the services pie primarily in the self-interests of the professions covered, not the clientele served. Unfortunately, there is little or no empirical evidence to support either position in a substantial way. Nonetheless, two of the most recent sets of regulations that cover MFT have gone the omnibus route—Virginia and Florida.

Williamson's (1979) article further questions the need for, and appropriateness of, regulatory measures related to marital and family therapy. Even the national boards of the American Association for Marriage and Family Therapy have taken stands on regulation that vacilate with the political winds going from active support and encouragement for legislation regulating MFTs to a "keeping the lid on" stance that seems to be a wait-and-see attitude recognizing current political realities. Focused work on marital and family therapy regulation is available in AAMFT's (1979) model legislation handbook. Additional insights into the general regulation dilemma may be gleaned from Hogan (1979).

CONCLUSION

Regulation of independent practice seems to be as much a result of the growing societal push for legal controls in many areas as it is a response to the needs of the citizens and the professions. In one respect this movement has been positive in that it has required the definition and outlining of professional practice in relation to what has existed, what exists, and what might exist. An outcome has been the emergence of interdisciplinary thinking regarding the provision of MFT services as well as interprofessional rivalry related to professional practice boundary disputes. Ethical and legal responsibilities have been delineated for the practitioner, and the individual finds it imperative to know and understand these regulations in relation to his or her practice.

The therapist can no longer practice whatever he or she wishes under the guise of an unregulated profession. Professional and legal responsibility for practice, as well as legal liability, is a fact of life. Not knowing about them is an illegitimate response; not abiding by the regulations poses not only illegal behavior but unprofessional and unethical conduct.

At this point the question of the regulation of family therapists cannot be posed in the "To be or not to be" format. The profession and the public already have been working on the issues and, at least in nine states, come to grips with the task. It would appear that the one constant to be dealt with is change in attitude, in regulation form, and in perceived need for a process of licensure or certification. The family therapist will need to keep constantly abreast of these changes to maintain the credentials necessary for practice. Involvement in the process, not a let-somebody-else-do-it attitude, will be essential if professional credibility is to be attained and continued.

Regulation of marital and family therapy can offer positive rewards to both the practitioner and the public. A cooperative venture would seem to be the needed direction of such efforts to serve the best interests of all concerned. Nevertheless, regulation is but one piece of the puzzle of professional competence and practice, and one must not lose sight of the whole.

REFERENCES

American Association for Marriage and Family Therapy. *Marital and family therapy: State licensing and certification model legislation.* Upland, Calif.: AAMFT, 1979.

California Association of Marriage and Family Therapists. *The California Therapist,* 1981, *10* (July/August), cover page. (Published by CAMFT, 2605 Camino del Rio South, Suite 200, San Diego, California 92108.)

Forster, J. Counselor credentialing revised. *The Personnel and Guidance Journal,* 1978, *56,* 593-598.

Fretz, B.R., & Mills, D.H. *Licensing and certification of psychologists and counselors.* San Francisco: Jossey-Bass, 1980.

Gross, S. The myth of professional licensing. *American Psychologist,* 1978, *33,* 1009-1016.

Hogan, D.B. *The regulation of psychotherapists (Vol. 2): A handbook of state licensure laws.* Cambridge, Mass.: Ballinger, 1979.

Nichols, W. *Marriage and family counseling: A legislative handbook.* Claremont, Calif.: American Association of Marriage and Family Counselors, 1974.

Olsen, L. Reflections on credentialing. *APA Monitor,* 1978, *9,* 3, 20.

Rutledge, A. State regulation of marriage counseling. *The Family Coordinator,* 1973, *22* 81-90.

Sporakowski, M.J., & Staniszewski, W.P. The regulation of marriage and family therapy: An update. *Journal of Marital and Family Therapy,* 1980, *6,* 335-348.

Williamson, D. State licensing—a necessary evil? *AAMFT Newsletter,* 1979, *10,* pp. 2, 5.